Signals and Communication Technology

This series is devoted to fundamentals and applications of modern methods of signal processing and cutting-edge communication technologies. The main topics are information and signal theory, acoustical signal processing, image processing and multimedia systems, mobile and wireless communications, and computer and communication networks. Volumes in the series address researchers in academia and industrial R&D departments. The series is application-oriented. The level of presentation of each individual volume, however, depends on the subject and can range from practical to scientific.

Indexing: All books in "Signals and Communication Technology" are indexed by Scopus and zbMATH

For general information about this book series, comments or suggestions, please contact Mary James at mary.james@springer.com or Ramesh Nath Premnath at ramesh.premnath@springer.com.

Sejal Shah · Rohit Thanki

Artificial Intelligence for Early Detection and Diagnosis of Lung Cancer

Springer

Sejal Shah
Department of Bioinformatics
Marwadi University
Rajkot, Gujarat, India

Rohit Thanki
IEEE
Rajkot, Gujarat, India

ISSN 1860-4862 ISSN 1860-4870 (electronic)
Signals and Communication Technology
ISBN 978-3-032-29614-6 ISBN 978-3-032-29615-3 (eBook)
https://doi.org/10.1007/978-3-032-29615-3

This Springer imprint is published by the registered company Springer Nature Switzerland AG
The registered company address is: Gewerbestrasse 11, 6330 Cham, Switzerland

Preface

The field of genomics has undergone a transformative evolution, driven by the convergence of high-throughput sequencing technologies and artificial intelligence (AI). This book explores the intersection of these two domains, offering a comprehensive overview of how AI is reshaping genomic research, precision medicine, and drug discovery. From foundational concepts to cutting-edge applications, the chapters delve into the technical, ethical, and regulatory dimensions of genomic AI.

Lung cancer remains the leading cause of cancer-related mortality worldwide, claiming approximately 1.8 million lives annually. Despite decades of progress in surgical, pharmacological, and radiotherapeutic interventions, survival rates remain low, largely because many cases are diagnosed at advanced stages when curative treatment options are limited. The convergence of artificial intelligence (AI) with medical imaging, clinical data analytics, and molecular oncology presents a transformative opportunity to reshape this trajectory through earlier detection, more precise diagnosis, and truly personalized treatment planning.

This book was conceived with a dual purpose: first, to provide clinicians, researchers, and students with a rigorous yet accessible foundation in lung cancer biology, staging, and the rapidly evolving landscape of AI-assisted diagnostics; and second, to document the design, implementation, and evaluation of a complete suite of AI diagnostic agents from individual specialist models to a fully integrated multimodal assessment system that together emulate the cognitive reasoning of a Multidisciplinary Team (MDT) tumor board.

The book is structured in two complementary parts. Chapters 1–4 establish the clinical and technological foundations: an introduction to lung cancer biology and risk factors; the classification, staging, and treatment landscape; the role of artificial intelligence in early detection; and a comprehensive review of current research trends including foundation models, federated learning, explainable AI, and large language models in oncological imaging. Chapters 5–8 present original applied research: Lung AI-Dx, an integrated multi-omics AI framework for NSCLC subtype classification, survival prediction, biomarker discovery, and drug repurposing; the Lung Cancer Risk Prediction (LCRP) Agent for clinical risk quantification; HieraLung and HistoLung, two complementary imaging AI agents for CT scan and histopathology analysis respectively; and the Multimodal Lung Cancer Assessment (MLCA) Agent, which orchestrates all three specialist agents and synthesizes their outputs using a generative AI model to produce a holistic diagnostic report.

A distinctive feature of this work is that it does not merely survey AI methods in the abstract, it builds, deploys, and evaluates them. Every agent documented in Chapters 6–8 is implemented as a functional Streamlit web application with downloadable HTML diagnostic reports, complete with annotated user interface screenshots, system architecture diagrams, class diagrams, data flow diagrams, and illustrative clinical cases. The datasets, model architectures, training protocols, and validation results are reported transparently to enable reproducibility and critical assessment.

This book is intended for a broad audience: oncologists and radiologists seeking to understand AI's diagnostic potential; computer scientists and biomedical engineers developing clinical decision support tools; postgraduate students in medical AI, bioinformatics, or digital health; and healthcare administrators evaluating AI adoption. No single-modality AI tool can replicate the integrative reasoning of an experienced clinical team, but a thoughtfully designed multimodal AI system can augment that reasoning, accelerate triage, and extend expert-level diagnostic support to settings where specialist access is limited.

We hope this book serves as both a practical reference and an inspiration for the next generation of AI-assisted healthcare systems.

Rajkot, India

Sejal Shah
Rohit Thanki

Acknowledgments Our task has been made easier and the final version of this book considerably improved thanks to the support we have received. We extend our heartfelt thanks to the publishing team for their invaluable guidance and encouragement during the creation of this book. We also wish to thank our colleagues and peers for their insightful discussions and contributions that enriched the content.

Competing Interests The authors have no competing interests to declare that are relevant to the content of this manuscript.

Contents

1 An Introduction to Lung Cancer ... 1
- 1.1 Introduction Related to Cancer and Its Treatment Methods ... 1
  - 1.1.1 History of Cancer ... 1
  - 1.1.2 Risk Factors for Cancer ... 3
  - 1.1.3 Classification of Cancer ... 4
  - 1.1.4 Types of Organs Cancer ... 6
  - 1.1.5 Cancer Diagnosis Methods ... 7
  - 1.1.6 Cancer Treatment Methods ... 9
- 1.2 Lung Anatomy ... 12
- 1.3 What is Lung Cancer? ... 14
- 1.4 Risk Factors for Lung Cancer ... 16
- 1.5 Prevention Against Lung Cancer ... 18
- 1.6 Summary ... 21
- References ... 21

2 Types, Diagnosis, and Treatment of Lung Cancer ... 23
- 2.1 Stages of Lung Cancer ... 23
  - 2.1.1 Stage 0 ... 24
  - 2.1.2 Stage I and Stage II ... 24
  - 2.1.3 Stage III ... 24
  - 2.1.4 Stage IV ... 25
- 2.2 Types of Lung Cancer ... 25
- 2.3 Early Detection of Lung Cancer ... 27
  - 2.3.1 Biopsies ... 27
  - 2.3.2 Imaging ... 28
- 2.4 Diagnosis of Lung Cancer ... 29
  - 2.4.1 Screening ... 30
  - 2.4.2 Staging ... 31
- 2.5 Treatment for Lung Cancer ... 33
  - 2.5.1 Surgery ... 33
  - 2.5.2 Chemotherapy ... 34

2.5.3 Radiation Therapy ... 36
2.5.4 Targeted Therapy ... 37
2.5.5 Immunotherapy ... 39
2.6 Summary ... 40
References ... 40

3 Artificial Intelligence and Its Role in Early Detection of Lung Cancer ... 43
3.1 Artificial Intelligence (AI) ... 43
3.2 AI in Healthcare Research ... 44
3.3 Role of AI in Cancer Detection ... 44
3.4 Roles of AI in Detection and Diagnosis of Lung Cancer ... 46
3.4.1 Automated Image Analysis ... 46
3.4.2 Computer-Aided Diagnosis (CAD) ... 46
3.4.3 Risk Stratification ... 46
3.4.4 Integration with Electronic Health Records (EHR) ... 47
3.4.5 Prediction Models ... 47
3.4.6 Mobile Health (mHealth) Solutions ... 48
3.5 Various Stages of Detection and Diagnosis of Lung Cancer Using AI ... 48
3.5.1 Screening and Triage ... 48
3.5.2 Histopathology Image Analysis ... 48
3.5.3 Prognosis and Risk Analysis ... 49
3.5.4 Treatment Planning and Response Monitoring ... 50
3.5.5 Clinical Decision Support ... 50
3.6 Summary ... 51
References ... 51

4 Current Research Trends for Early Screening of Lung Cancer Using AI ... 55
4.1 Overview of Research Trends ... 55
4.2 Foundation Models and Large-Scale Pre-training ... 56
4.3 Multimodal AI Fusion ... 57
4.4 Federated Learning for Privacy-Preserving Multi-site AI ... 58
4.5 Self-supervised and Contrastive Learning ... 58
4.6 Transformer Architectures in Lung Cancer Imaging ... 59
4.7 Explainable AI (XAI) in Lung Cancer Screening ... 60
4.8 AI-Augmented Liquid Biopsy ... 60
4.9 Large Language Models and AI-Assisted Radiology Reporting ... 61
4.10 Performance Benchmarking of Recent AI Models ... 61
4.11 Challenges and Limitations ... 62
4.12 Future Directions ... 62
4.13 Summary ... 62
References ... 63

5 LungAI-Dx: An Integrated AI Framework for Molecular Subtype Classification, Survival Prediction, and Precision Oncology in Non-small Cell Lung Cancer 65
5.1 Introduction 65
5.1.1 Global Burden of Lung Cancer 65
5.1.2 NSCLC Subtypes and Clinical Significance 66
5.1.3 Artificial Intelligence in Molecular Oncology: Background 66
5.1.4 Objectives and Chapter Organization 67
5.2 Datasets and Data Sources 67
5.2.1 Gene Expression Data (NCBI GEO) 67
5.2.2 TCGA Clinical and Genomic Data 68
5.2.3 Class Distribution and Imbalance Analysis 68
5.3 Methodology 69
5.3.1 Feature Engineering and Selection 69
5.3.2 Class Imbalance Correction: BorderlineSMOTE-2 69
5.3.3 Machine Learning Classification Models 70
5.3.4 Hyperparameter Optimization with Optuna 70
5.3.5 Survival Analysis Methods 70
5.3.6 Multi-omics Integration Strategies 71
5.3.7 Biomarker Discovery and Drug Repurposing 71
5.4 Results and Discussion 71
5.4.1 Classification Performance 72
5.4.2 Survival Analysis Results 76
5.4.3 Biomarker Discovery Results 80
5.4.4 Multi-omics Integration Results 82
5.4.5 Drug Repurposing and Therapeutic Recommendations 85
5.4.6 Clinical Risk Assessment Models 85
5.5 LungAI-Dx Clinical Decision-Support Platform 86
5.6 Limitations and Future Directions 91
5.6.1 Limitations 92
5.6.2 Future Directions 93
5.7 Summary 93
References 94

6 The Lung Cancer Risk Prediction (LCRP) Agent 97
6.1 Introduction and Clinical Motivation 97
6.2 System Architecture 98
6.3 Patient Input Features 98
6.4 Model Development and Comparative Evaluation 98
6.5 User Interface of LCRP Agent 98
6.5.1 Patient Data Entry Interface 98

6.5.2 Post-Prediction Interface and Risk Assessment Result Display 100
6.6 Generated Report 100
6.7 Summary 103
References 105

7 CT and Histopathology Imaging AI Agents: HieraLung and HistoLung 107
7.1 Introduction to HieraLung 107
7.2 System Architecture and Pipeline 108
7.2.1 Application Flowchart 108
7.2.2 Data Flow Diagram 108
7.3 Dataset Used for Development of HieraLung Agent 108
7.4 CNN Model Architecture and Performance 111
7.5 User Interface of HieraLung Agent 113
7.5.1 Landing Screen 113
7.5.2 Post-upload State 114
7.5.3 Post-prediction Results 114
7.5.4 Report Download State 115
7.6 Generated HieraLung Report 116
7.7 Introduction to HistoLung 116
7.8 System Architecture and Pipeline 118
7.9 Dataset Used for Development of HistoLung Agent 118
7.10 CNN Model Architecture and Performance for HistoLung Agent 118
7.11 User Interface of HieraLung Agent 121
7.11.1 Landing Screen 121
7.11.2 Post-upload State 122
7.11.3 Post-prediction Results 122
7.11.4 Report Download State 122
7.12 Generated HistoLung Report 123
7.13 Summary 124
References 125

8 The Multi-modal Lung Cancer Assessment (MLCA) Agent 127
8.1 Introduction and Clinical Motivation 127
8.2 System Architecture 127
8.3 Class Diagram for Object-Oriented Design 129
8.4 Data Flow and Sequence Diagrams 131
8.5 Two-Stage Processing Pipeline 132
8.5.1 Stage 1: Parallel Specialized AI Analysis 133
8.5.2 Stage 2: Generative AI Synthesis 134
8.6 User Interface of MLCA Agent 134
8.6.1 Landing Screen 134
8.6.2 Post-Upload State, All Three Files Loaded 135
8.6.3 Post-Analysis Results 1 (Three AI Analysis) 136

8.6.4 Post-Analysis Results 2 (Holistic AI Report) 136
8.7 Generated Report of Multi-modal Lung Cancer Analysis Report 136
8.8 Illustrative Case Results and Cross-Modality Concordance 137
8.9 Clinical Value, Limitations, and Future Directions 139
8.10 Summary 140
References 140

Index 141

List of Figures

Fig. 1.1 Anatomy of the human respiratory system 12
Fig. 3.1 Generalized AI-enabled workflow for cancer detection 45
Fig. 3.2 Sequential stages of AI-assisted lung cancer detection and diagnosis 49
Fig. 4.1 Integrated AI-driven screening workflow 56
Fig. 4.2 Self-supervised learning architecture for foundation models 57
Fig. 4.3 Architecture of the lightweight hybrid foundation model (LHFM) 58
Fig. 4.4 Federated learning workflow with secure aggregation 59
Fig. 4.5 Vision transformer self-attention heatmap 60
Fig. 5.1 Comparative performance of all five classifiers across test-set evaluation metrics 73
Fig. 5.2 ROC curves for all five classifiers on the test set (one-vs-rest per class) 73
Fig. 5.3 XGBoost confusion matrix on the held-out test set 74
Fig. 5.4 Per-class one-vs-rest AUC heatmap comparing all five classifiers 75
Fig. 5.5 Heatmap of the top 50 most discriminative transcriptomic features 75
Fig. 5.6 Kaplan–Meier overall survival curve for the TCGA-NSCLC cohort 76
Fig. 5.7 Kaplan–Meier survival curves stratified by AJCC pathological stage (I–IV). Log-rank $p < 0.0001$. Stage IV patients had no 5-year survivors in this cohort 77
Fig. 5.8 Cox proportional hazards' model forest plot 79
Fig. 5.9 Kaplan–Meier survival curves for low-, intermediate-, and high-risk Prognostic Index groups 79
Fig. 5.10 Somatic mutation landscape across the TCGA-LUAD and TCGA-LUSC cohort 80
Fig. 5.11 Tumor mutational burden (TMB) distribution by cancer subtype 81

Fig. 5.12 Immune cell deconvolution heatmap across all samples 83
Fig. 5.13 DNA methylation landscape across TCGA-NSCLC samples 83
Fig. 5.14 Multi-omics integration strategy comparison, AUC achieved by each of the four strategies 84
Fig. 5.15 Drug-gene interaction network for NSCLC driver genes 85
Fig. 5.16 LungAI-Dx Dashboard, **a** main landing page with platform summary statistics, 14-stage pipeline overview, and key clinical facts reference tab, **b** Platform Modules overview with nine interactive module cards and embedded Figures Gallery showing key analytical visualizations, **c** Figures Gallery continuation with key analytical visualizations and Research Use Only (RUO) disclaimer 88
Fig. 5.17 Lung Subtype Prediction Module **a** manual feature entry input interface for 9904 Affymetrix probe expression values with three input modes (manual, CSV upload, random sample), **b** prediction results displaying predicted class (Normal) with calibrated class probability bar chart, **c** SHAP explanation showing the top 3 transcriptomic features driving the individual classification decision with directional SHAP values 89
Fig. 5.18 Clinical risk assessment module **a** clinical parameter input interface with age, pathological stage, smoking pack-years, gender, cancer type, and ECOG performance status controls, **b** results showing risk scores, stage category, overall risk tier (LOW RISK), donut chart visualizations, and evidence-based clinical recommendations 90
Fig. 5.19 Survival Prediction Module, individual patient survival estimate showing clinical input parameters, Prognostic Index (PI) group assignment (intermediate risk), Cox linear predictor value, estimated median OS, and personalized survival curve with confidence interval 91
Fig. 5.20 Drug recommendations module **a** patient biomarker profile input interface with actionable mutation checkboxes, TMB, PD-L1 TPS, and treatment context parameters, **b** output displaying 8 prioritized FDA-approved agents with biomarker targets, mechanisms of action, treatment settings, and pivotal clinical trial references 92
Fig. 6.1 LCRP agent patient data entry interface **a** upper section of the LCRP agent patient input form. Demographic and primary symptom fields with slider and dropdown widgets **b** lower section of the LCRP Agent patient input form, with remaining risk factor fields, 'Analyze Patient Data' button, and educational disclaimer 101

Fig. 6.2 LCRP agent post-prediction interface and risk assessment result **a** LCRP agent input form in post-prediction state. All entered values preserved for audit. Default profile: Age 50, Male, non-smoker, SpO_2 95%, energy level 50%. **b** LCRP agent risk assessment result: Risk category = low, predicted risk = 6.00%. Download full report button visible ... 102
Fig. 6.3 Generated LCRP agent lung cancer risk prediction report 104
Fig. 7.1 HieraLung application flowchart: two-stage hierarchical diagnostic logic gating subtype classification on malignancy detection ... 109
Fig. 7.2 HieraLung 12-step data flow sequence diagram (User → UI → Agent → Models) ... 110
Fig. 7.3 HieraLung landing screen ... 114
Fig. 7.4 HieraLung post-CT upload state ... 115
Fig. 7.5 HieraLung post-diagnosis results ... 115
Fig. 7.6 HieraLung report download state ... 116
Fig. 7.7 HieraLung diagnostic report (HTML) ... 117
Fig. 7.8 HistoLung application flowchart: linear six-step pipeline from histopathology image upload to diagnostic result display ... 119
Fig. 7.9 HistoLung 8-step data flow sequence diagram (User, UI, Agent, Model) ... 120
Fig. 7.10 HistoLung landing screen ... 121
Fig. 7.11 HistoLung post-upload state ... 122
Fig. 7.12 HistoLung post-diagnosis results ... 123
Fig. 7.13 HistoLung report download state ... 123
Fig. 7.14 HistoLung diagnostic report (HTML) ... 124
Fig. 8.1 MLCA agent system architecture: three parallel input modalities → three specialized AI modules → generative AI synthesis → comprehensive diagnostic report ... 128
Fig. 8.2 MLCA agent application-level diagram. Streamlit server logic orchestrates LCRP, HieraLung, HistoLung agents and report generation module (external generative AI API) 129
Fig. 8.3 MLCA agent deployment: HTTPS → Python backend on Cloud/VM → local AI model files (LCRP.joblib; HieraLung.h5; HistoLung.h5) + external generative AI API ... 129
Fig. 8.4 MLCA agent UML class diagram. Streamlit App orchestrates LCRP Agent, HieraLung Agent, HistoLung agent, and report generator (which uses generative AI client) ... 130
Fig. 8.5 MLCA agent data flow: three parallel Stage 1 pipelines converge into a JSON prompt for Generative AI synthesis, producing the comprehensive diagnostic report ... 131
Fig. 8.6 MLCA agent 12-step sequence diagram. Steps 1–7: data upload and parallel specialist agent analysis. Steps 8–12: LLM synthesis and report delivery ... 131

Fig. 8.7 MLCA Agent landing screen 135
Fig. 8.8 MLCA Agent post-upload state 135
Fig. 8.9 MLCA Agent three-panel analysis results 136
Fig. 8.10 MLCA Agent holistic AI-generated report 137
Fig. 8.11 MLCA Agent downloaded HTML report 138

List of Tables

Table 3.1	Core AI components and their applications in medicine	44
Table 3.2	AI applications across healthcare research domains	45
Table 3.3	Landmark computer-aided diagnosis (CAD) systems for lung cancer	47
Table 3.4	AI roles across the lung cancer detection and management continuum	50
Table 4.1	Comparison of traditional and AI-augmented lung cancer screening	56
Table 4.2	Diagnostic and prognostic performance of the UCLIF foundation model	57
Table 4.3	Performance gains through multimodal data fusion strategies	58
Table 4.4	Federated learning models and privacy-preserving protocols	59
Table 4.5	Benchmarking vision transformer architectures in lung cancer classification	59
Table 4.6	Comparison of explainable AI (XAI) methodologies	60
Table 4.7	Performance and utilities of AI-augmented liquid biopsy biomarkers	61
Table 4.8	Performance comparison of AI models versus human radiologists	61
Table 5.1	GEO gene expression datasets used for NSCLC classification	68
Table 5.2	Fivefold stratified cross-validation performance (training set)	72
Table 5.3	Test set classification performance, all models	72
Table 5.4	Per-class classification report, XGBoost best model (test set)	74
Table 5.5	Kaplan–Meier overall survival statistics (TCGA cohort)	77
Table 5.6	Stage-stratified 5-year overall survival (TCGA-NSCLC cohort)	78

Table 5.7 Cox proportional hazards' multivariable model results 78
Table 5.8 Prognostic Index (PI) risk group stratification 80
Table 5.9 Driver gene mutation frequencies in TCGA-LUAD and TCGA-LUSC 81
Table 5.10 Tumor mutational burden and immunotherapy eligibility 82
Table 5.11 DNA methylation landscape statistics (TCGA-NSCLC cohort) 83
Table 5.12 Multi-omics integration strategy comparison, classification AUC 84
Table 5.13 Immunotherapy eligibility by biomarker threshold 86
Table 5.14 Auxiliary clinical risk model performance (TCGA clinical dataset) 86
Table 5.15 LungAI-Dx Streamlit application module summary 87
Table 6.1 Patient input features collected by the LCRP agent 99
Table 6.2 MLOps model comparison: random forest, gradient boosting, XGBoost 99
Table 6.3 Per-class classification report for all three models (test set) ... 100
Table 6.4 Risk category classification scheme 100
Table 7.1 Balanced IQ-OTH/NCCD dataset summary for HieraLung triage model (LC_Cases_Classifier) training and validation 110
Table 7.2 Balanced chest CT scan images dataset summary for HieraLung subtype model (LC_Types_Classifier) training and validation 111
Table 7.3 CNN architecture used by HieraLung triage model, total trainable parameters: 51,475,523 112
Table 7.4 CNN architecture used by HieraLung subtype model, total trainable parameters: 51,476,036 112
Table 7.5 Validation-set classification reports for LC cases classifier 113
Table 7.6 HieraLung diagnostic output categories and clinical action guidance 114
Table 7.7 CNN_LC_Histo_Classifier architecture, total trainable parameters: 51,475,523 120
Table 7.8 CNN_LC_Histo_Classifier training and validation report 121
Table 8.1 All six classes in the MLCA agent object model 130
Table 8.2 Detailed 12-step interaction flow for the MLCA agent 132
Table 8.3 Three parallel Stage 1 specialized analysis pipelines 133
Table 8.4 Five core tasks performed by the generative AI model in Stage 2 of the MLCA Agent 133
Table 8.5 Illustrative case results 139

Chapter 1
An Introduction to Lung Cancer

1.1 Introduction Related to Cancer and Its Treatment Methods

Cancer is a broad group of diseases characterized by the uncontrolled growth and spread of abnormal cells [1]. It is one of the leading causes of death worldwide, responsible for roughly one in five deaths globally [1]. In 2020 alone, an estimated 19.3 million new cancer cases were diagnosed and 10.0 million people died from cancer across the world [2]. These numbers highlight the immense global burden of cancer and underscore the importance of understanding its causes, classification, diagnosis, and treatment. In this section, we introduce general concepts about cancer, laying the groundwork for a focused discussion on lung cancer in the later sections.

1.1.1 History of Cancer

The history of cancer extends back to ancient times. The earliest known description of cancer appears in ancient Egyptian manuscripts. The Edwin Smith Papyrus (circa 3000 BC) described tumors (likely breast cancer) as an "incurable" swelling [3]. Similarly, the Ebers Papyrus (~ 1500 BC) recorded cases of tumors of the skin, stomach, rectum, and uterus [1]. In these early texts, disease was often attributed to divine causes, and treatments were limited to crude methods like cautery or pastes [1]. It wasn't until around 400 BC that the Greek physician Hippocrates provided a more scientific description. He coined the term "karkinos" (crab) to describe malignancies, which is the origin of the word cancer. Hippocrates believed cancer was caused by an imbalance of bodily humors (particularly an excess of black bile). His school distinguished between benign and malignant tumors and suggested treatments such as surgery, if possible, though truly malignant cases were deemed incurable at the time. The Roman physician Galen later expanded on the humoral theory, also attributing

S. Shah and R. Thanki, *Artificial Intelligence for Early Detection and Diagnosis of Lung Cancer*, Signals and Communication Technology,
https://doi.org/10.1007/978-3-032-29615-3_1

incurable cancers to excess black bile [1]. These early ideas, while incorrect in mechanism, marked the first attempts to systematically understand cancer.

After the ancient period, progress was slow for many centuries. There are sparse records of cancer treatment in the medieval era aside from surgical removal of visible growths and folk remedies. Significant advances began in the eighteenth and nineteenth centuries. In 1775, British surgeon Percivall Pott observed a link between chimney soot exposure and scrotal cancer in chimney sweeps—the first clear evidence that environmental factors could cause cancer [1]. This was a landmark in recognizing carcinogens (cancer-causing agents) and the concept of cancer prevention by avoiding exposures. By the mid-nineteenth century, scientists like Rudolph Virchow were studying cancer under the microscope, discovering abnormal cells and coining terms like leukemia [4]. The late 1800s also saw technical breakthroughs: Wilhelm Röntgen's discovery of X-rays in 1895 enabled physicians to visualize tumors inside the body, and in 1898 Marie and Pierre Curie discovered radium, which led to the first radiation therapy for cancer shortly thereafter. Surgery for cancer became more systematic as well for example, the first radical mastectomy for breast cancer was performed in 1882 [4]. These developments laid the foundation for modern cancer diagnosis and treatment.

The twentieth century brought an explosion of knowledge about cancer biology and therapy. Researchers realized cancer is fundamentally a disease of cell mutation and uncontrolled division [1]. The first chemotherapy drugs were introduced in the 1940s; for instance, antimetabolites like aminopterin induced remissions in childhood leukemia [4], and the first alkylating agent (nitrogen mustard) was approved in 1949. In 1950, studies by Doll and Hill and others conclusively linked cigarette smoking to lung cancer, establishing tobacco as a powerful carcinogen[4]. The subsequent decades saw combination chemotherapy regimens that dramatically improved survival for diseases like leukemia, the advent of hormonal therapies (e.g., antiestrogen treatment for breast cancer in the 1970s), and later targeted therapies that home in on specific molecular abnormalities of cancer cells (such as the drug imatinib targeting the Philadelphia chromosome in chronic myeloid leukemia). By the late twentieth and early twenty-first centuries, immunotherapy emerged, treatments that stimulate the patient's immune system to attack cancer fulfilling ideas first hinted at by researchers like William Coley in the 1890s [1]. Today, cancer research spans everything from genetics to personalized medicine. In summary, our understanding of cancer has evolved from mystical explanations to a detailed scientific picture: we now know cancer is not a single disease but over 100 distinct diseases, each with specific causes and behaviors, and we have a broad arsenal of treatments ranging from surgery and radiation to advanced drugs. This historical journey underpins current approaches to cancer care.

1.1.2 Risk Factors for Cancer

Cancer does not have a single cause; it arises from a complex interplay of genetic and environmental factors. However, researchers have identified many key risk factors that increase the likelihood of developing cancer. These can be grouped into several categories:

- **Lifestyle Factors**: Certain lifestyle choices are strongly linked to cancer risk. Chief among these is tobacco use smoking is the single largest preventable cause of cancer worldwide [1]. It is implicated not only in lung cancer but also in cancers of the mouth, throat, esophagus, bladder, and others. Heavy alcohol consumption is another lifestyle factor associated with cancers such as liver, esophagus, and breast. Diet and body weight also play a role: for example, obesity and diets high in processed/red meats have been linked to higher rates of colorectal and other cancers [1]. Conversely, a healthy diet rich in fruits and vegetables and regular physical activity can modestly reduce risk. Lack of exercise and chronic inflammation (as seen in obesity) are thought to contribute to cancer development. In summary, lifestyle-related factors (smoking, alcohol, diet, exercise) are estimated to account for a large proportion of cancers; one UK study attributed nearly 4 in 10 cancer cases in 2015 to such modifiable factors (with smoking being the top contributor) [1].
- **Environmental and Occupational Exposures**: Many cancers are triggered by long-term exposure to carcinogens in our environment. For instance, ionizing radiation (from sources like ultraviolet sunlight or medical X-rays) can damage DNA and lead to skin cancer or leukemias. Repeated exposure to chemicals is also a risk classic examples include asbestos (linked to mesothelioma and lung cancer), benzene (linked to leukemia), and arsenic (linked to skin, lung, and bladder cancers). People in certain occupations may encounter higher levels of carcinogens (industrial chemicals, coal tar, diesel exhaust, etc.) and thus have elevated cancer risks [1, 4]. Air pollution is another environmental factor: inhalation of fine particulate matter or other pollutants over years can increase lung cancer incidence [1]. Infections can be considered environmental factors as well as several pathogens that are known to cause cancer. For example, human papillomavirus (HPV) causes cervical cancer, hepatitis B and C viruses cause liver cancer, and Helicobacter pylori infection in the stomach can lead to gastric cancer. Collectively, infections account for a significant share of cancers in some regions. Public health initiatives like vaccination against HPV and hepatitis B are therefore also cancer prevention measures.
- **Genetic Predisposition**: A person's genetic makeup can influence their susceptibility to cancer. Most cancers are not purely hereditary, but having a family history of certain cancers can increase risk. For example, individuals with a first-degree relative (parent or sibling) who had cancer may be at higher risk of developing that cancer themselves [3]. In some cases, this is due to inherited mutations in specific genes. Well-known examples include mutations in BRCA1/2 genes that greatly raise the risk of breast and ovarian cancer, or mutations in mismatch repair

genes that cause Lynch syndrome and increase colon cancer risk. These inherited syndromes are relatively rare but significant. More commonly, genetic risk comes from a combination of many small-effect variants plus shared family lifestyle. It's estimated that lung cancer, having a close relative with the disease confers about a 1.5-fold increase in risk [5]. While we cannot change our genes, this knowledge helps identify high-risk individuals who might benefit from enhanced screening or preventive measures.

It is important to emphasize that having one or more risk factors does not guarantee someone will get cancer, it only increases the probability. Likewise, some people develop cancer without any known risk factors. Cancer causation is multi-factorial and often involves an accumulation of risks over time (age itself is a major risk factor, as most cancers occur in older adults). Understanding these risk factors allows for preventive strategies, such as lifestyle modifications and reducing exposures, which can significantly lower the overall cancer burden in the population.

1.1.3 Classification of Cancer

Because cancer is not a single disease, doctors and scientists classify cancer in several ways to describe and understand them. The three common classification schemes are by histologic type, by organ/site of origin, and by molecular features:

- **Classification by Tissue (Histological Type)**: One way to categorize cancer is by the type of tissue and cells from which it arises [6]. Under this scheme, there are five major histological categories of cancer:
  - **Carcinomas**: Cancers arising from epithelial cells (the cells that line body surfaces, glands, and organs). Carcinomas are by far the most common type of cancer, accounting for about 80–90% of all cancer cases [6]. Examples include lung cancer, breast cancer, colon cancer, and prostate cancer, since these organs are lined with epithelial tissue. Carcinomas are further sub-classified, for example into adenocarcinomas (from glandular or mucus-secreting epithelium) and squamous cell carcinomas (from flat epithelial cells) [6].
  - **Sarcomas**: Cancers arising from connective or supportive tissues, such as bone, muscle, fat, cartilage, or fibrous tissue [6]. Sarcomas are relatively rare. Examples include osteosarcoma (bone cancer), leiomyosarcoma (smooth muscle), and liposarcoma (fat) [6]. Sarcomas are often present as tumors of the limbs or trunk and can occur in younger age groups compared to carcinomas.
  - **Leukemias**: Cancers of the blood or bone marrow, characterized by the overproduction of abnormal white blood cells. Unlike most other cancers, leukemias generally do not form solid tumors; instead, cancer cells circulate in the blood ("liquid cancers") [6]. Leukemia can cause symptoms like anemia, infection, and bleeding due to bone marrow failure.

- **Lymphomas and Myeloma**: These are cancers of the immune system cells. Lymphomas are cancers of lymphocytes (a type of white blood cell) that typically present as solid tumors in lymph nodes or other lymphatic tissues [7]. They are divided into Hodgkin lymphoma and non-Hodgkin lymphoma. Multiple myeloma is a cancer of plasma cells (antibody-producing cells in the bone marrow) [6]. It often leads to bone pain, anemia, and kidney problems.
- **Mixed and Other Types**: Some cancers have mixed characteristics. For example, carcinosarcomas have both carcinoma and sarcoma components, and adenosquamous carcinoma has both glandular and squamous features [7]. There are also embryonal tumors known as blastomas (e.g., neuroblastoma, retinoblastoma) that arise from precursor cells and are more common in children. These represent a small fraction of cancers but underscore that tumors can defy simple classification when they contain multiple cell types.

• **Classification by Organ or Primary Site**: Another common way to classify cancer is by its site of origin in the body (organ-based classification). For instance, we speak of lung cancer, breast cancer, colorectal cancer, prostate cancer, skin cancer, and so on, based on where the tumor started. This organ-based naming is used in clinical practice because cancers of the same organ often share similarities in symptoms and treatment. It is important to note that the organ name (e.g., "lung cancer") often implicitly refers to the most common histologic type in that organ (lung cancers are usually carcinomas of the bronchial epithelium). Organ-based classification is intuitive for patients and healthcare providers—for example, a "liver cancer" workup or clinic is focused on tumors in the liver, whether they are hepatocellular carcinomas or another type. Many cancers also spread (metastasize) to other organs, but they are still classified by their site of origin (a breast cancer that spread to bone is not "bone cancer," it is metastatic breast cancer). Organ classification is closely tied to screening guidelines (for instance, colonoscopy to detect colon cancer) and specialist care (e.g., gynecologic oncologists treat cervical and ovarian cancers).
• **Classification by Molecular Features**: In recent years, our understanding of cancer at the molecular level has led to a more refined classification based on genetic and biochemical characteristics of the tumor. Cancers that look identical under the microscope may have very different gene mutations or protein markers that affect how they behave and respond to treatment. For example, breast cancers are often classified by the presence or absence of hormone receptors (ER, PR) and HER2 protein labels that guide therapy decisions. Lung cancers can be tested for mutations in genes like EGFR, ALK, or KRAS, which identify subsets of tumors that may respond to specific targeted drugs. This molecular classification is becoming increasingly important: it allows for "personalized medicine" where treatment is tailored to the genetic makeup of the cancer. It also sometimes reveals relationships between cancers of different organs for instance, a rare mutation might be found in both a colon cancer and a stomach cancer, suggesting they could be treated with the same targeted therapy even though they arise from different sites [8]. While traditional pathology remains fundamental for diagnosis,

these molecular sub-classifications add another layer that is especially relevant for modern targeted and immune therapies.

In summary, cancer classification can be viewed on three levels, what the cells look like (histology), where the cancer started (organ site), and what key molecular abnormalities it carries. All three classification methods are used in concert to guide diagnosis and treatment.

1.1.4 Types of Organs Cancer

Cancers can arise in virtually any organ of the body. However, a few major organ-specific cancers account for a large proportion of the global cancer burden. In terms of frequency, the most diagnosed cancers worldwide are those of the breast, lung, colon/rectum, prostate, and stomach [2]. For the first time in recent statistics, female breast cancer has become the most commonly occurring cancer globally (by number of new cases), followed closely by lung cancer, then colorectal cancer, prostate cancer, and stomach cancer [2]. Each of these cancers originates in a different organ and has distinct risk factors and disease characteristics:

- **Breast Cancer**: A malignancy of breast tissue, most often arising from the lining of milk ducts (ductal carcinoma). It is the leading cancer in women worldwide, accounting for about 1 in 8 cancer diagnoses [2]. Improved awareness and screening (e.g., mammography) have led to many breast cancers being caught early, and treatments like hormone therapy have significantly improved survival in many cases. Risk factors include hormonal factors, certain genetic mutations (like BRCA genes), and lifestyle factors (alcohol intake, obesity).
- **Lung Cancer**: Cancer arising in the lung, usually in the bronchial lining of the airways. Lung cancer is the leading cause of cancer death globally for both men and women [9]. This is largely due to its aggressive nature and the fact that it is often diagnosed at a late stage. The primary risk factor is tobacco smoking (present in many cases), although non-smokers can also develop lung cancer, especially certain subtypes. Lung cancer's global impact is huge in 2022; it was estimated that about 2.5 million people were diagnosed with lung cancer and over 1.8 million died from it [9]. We will discuss lung cancer in detail in subsequent sections of this chapter.
- **Colorectal Cancer**: Cancer of the colon or rectum (often grouped together due to their anatomical proximity). It is a common cancer in both men and women worldwide (typically the third most common in incidence). Colorectal cancer often begins as a benign polyp that can turn cancerous over time. Diets high in red and processed meats, low physical activity, obesity, and age are important risk factors. Screening methods like colonoscopy can detect and remove precancerous polyps, thereby preventing colorectal cancer or catching it at an early, curable stage.
- **Prostate Cancer**: A cancer of the prostate gland (found only in men), and one of the most frequently diagnosed cancers in men (especially in developed countries).

Many prostate cancers grow slowly and may not cause harm in a man's lifetime, but others are more aggressive. Risk increases with age, and there are disparities in incidence and outcomes among different ethnic groups (with African ancestry men at higher risk). PSA blood tests and improved imaging are used for early detection, though screening approaches vary internationally due to concerns of overdiagnosis.

- **Stomach (Gastric) Cancer**: Once among the top causes of cancer death globally, stomach cancer remains common, particularly in East Asia and parts of Latin America. It is often linked to chronic infection with Helicobacter pylori bacteria in the stomach, as well as dietary factors like high salt intake and preserved foods. Incidence has declined in some regions thanks to refrigeration (less need for salted foods) and H. pylori treatment. Stomach cancer often presents late with symptoms like weight loss and persistent stomach pain.

Other significant organ cancers include liver cancer (often related to hepatitis B/C infection or alcohol abuse), cervical cancer (caused by HPV infection, a major cause of cancer death in women in low-resource countries, though largely preventable by vaccination and Pap smear screening), esophageal cancer, pancreatic cancer, kidney cancer, bladder cancer, melanoma of the skin, and non-melanoma skin cancers (the latter are extremely common but usually less lethal). Each organ cancer has its own profile of risk factors and clinical behavior. For example, pancreatic cancer is notorious for late presentation and poor prognosis, whereas thyroid cancer is often very treatable.

1.1.5 Cancer Diagnosis Methods

Early and accurate diagnosis of cancer is crucial for effective treatment. A variety of methods and tools are used to detect cancer and determine its extent:

- **Imaging Tests**: Medical imaging is a cornerstone of cancer diagnosis and staging. Techniques such as X-rays, ultrasound, computed tomography (CT) scans, magnetic resonance imaging (MRI), and positron emission tomography (PET) scans allow doctors to visualize masses or abnormalities inside the body [9]. For example, a chest X-ray might reveal a suspicious nodule in the lung, or an MRI might show a brain tumor. Imaging helps locate the tumor, measure its size, and check for spread (metastasis) to other organs (such as using bone scans to look for cancer in bones). Each imaging modality has specific uses: CT scans provide detailed cross-sectional views and are often used for cancers of the chest, abdomen, and pelvis; MRIs are excellent for soft tissue detail (e.g., brain, spinal cord); PET scans can highlight metabolically active cancer cells throughout the body. Imaging is noninvasive and is also used to monitor response to treatment.
- **Endoscopic Examinations**: For certain organs, doctors use endoscopes, thin, flexible tubes with cameras to look inside the body directly. Examples include colonoscopy (to detect colon polyps or colon cancer), gastroscopy (to view the

stomach for ulcers or tumors), bronchoscopy (to inspect the airways and lungs for tumors), and laparoscopy (surgical endoscopy to inspect the abdomen). Endoscopies not only visualize suspicious areas, but they also allow for taking tissue samples (biopsies) on the spot if needed.

- **Biopsy and Pathological Analysis**: Biopsy, the removal of a small sample of tissue for examination is the definitive way to diagnose cancer. Imaging tests may suggest a tumor is present, but only microscopic analysis of tissue can confirm if it is cancer and determine the type. Depending on the location, biopsies can be done with a needle (fine needle aspiration or core needle biopsy), an endoscopic tool, or surgical excision. In the laboratory, a pathologist examines the tissue under a microscope to identify cancer cells. Normal cells are uniform and organized, whereas cancer cells often appear irregular, vary in size and shape, and show chaotic arrangement [10]. The pathologist's report will typically provide the cancer's type (e.g., squamous cell carcinoma), grade (how abnormal the cells look, which hints at aggressiveness), and other features. In many cases, "in most situations, a biopsy is the only way to definitively diagnose cancer" [10] this underscores its importance. Modern pathology may also include immunohistochemistry or molecular testing on biopsy to further classify the cancer.
- **Laboratory Tests and Tumor Markers**: Routine lab tests can sometimes give clues to cancer. For instance, a complete blood count (CBC) might show abnormal white cell counts in leukemia [10]. Blood chemistry may reveal organ dysfunction caused by cancer spread (like elevated liver enzymes if liver is involved). More specific are tumor markers substances produced by cancer cells (or by the body in response to cancer) that can be detected in blood or other body fluids. Examples include prostate-specific antigen (PSA) for prostate cancer, CA-125 for ovarian cancer, alpha-fetoprotein (AFP) for liver cancer, and carcinoembryonic antigen (CEA) for colon cancer. Tumor markers can aid in diagnosis and are often used to monitor treatment response or detect recurrence, but most are not definitive enough to use for screening the general population (because they can be elevated in non-cancerous conditions too). Advances in molecular biology have also led to liquid biopsies, where blood tests detect circulating tumor DNA or cells shed by tumors; these are emerging tools for diagnosis and monitoring.
- **Genetic and Molecular Testing**: Increasingly, if cancer is confirmed, additional tests are done on the tumor tissue (or sometimes blood) to look for specific genetic mutations, chromosomal changes, or protein expression levels. These tests are critical for certain cancers to guide therapy. For example, breast cancer biopsies are tested for estrogen receptors and HER2 status; lung adenocarcinomas might be tested for EGFR or ALK mutations. The results can determine if targeted therapy or immunotherapy is likely to be effective. Molecular testing can also identify hereditary cancer syndromes by finding germline mutations (for instance, testing a young breast cancer patient for a BRCA mutation to guide family counseling).

In practice, diagnosing a suspected cancer often involves a combination of these methods. For example, consider a patient with a persistent cough, they might get a chest CT scan (imaging) that shows a lung mass, then undergo a bronchoscopy or needle biopsy to obtain tissue, which is examined by pathology for a definitive diagnosis, and the cancer cells might be tested for certain mutations. Once a cancer is diagnosed, additional imaging (CT, PET, MRI, etc.) is usually done to stage the cancer (determine how far it has spread). Staging is commonly described by the TNM system (Tumor size, Node involvement, Metastasis) and grouped into stages I through IV [7]. Accurate staging guides treatment decisions and helps predict prognosis. Overall, the modern approach to cancer diagnosis is comprehensive and multidisciplinary, aiming to detect cancer as early as possible and characterize them in detail to inform optimal management.

1.1.6 Cancer Treatment Methods

Once cancer is diagnosed, a treatment plan must be devised. Cancer treatment is highly individualized, based on the type of cancer, its stage, and the patient's health and preferences. Common cancer treatment methods include:

- **Surgery**: Surgical removal of the tumor is one of the oldest and most effective cancer treatments. The goal of surgery is to excise the cancer completely (with a margin of normal tissue) if possible [10]. Surgery is often the first-line treatment for localized cancers that have not spread, such as early-stage breast cancer, colon cancer, or lung cancer. In some cases (e.g., breast cancer), minimally invasive surgeries or organ-sparing surgeries can be done. Surgery can also be used for diagnosis (surgical biopsy) or for palliation (e.g., removing part of a tumor that's causing pain or obstruction even if the cancer isn't curable). Advances in surgical techniques, like laparoscopic and robotic surgery, have reduced recovery time and complications.
- **Radiation Therapy**: This treatment uses high-energy radiation (such as X-rays, gamma rays, or proton beams) to kill cancer cells or damage them so they cannot grow. Radiation can be delivered externally by a machine (external beam radiation) or internally by placing radioactive sources into or near the tumor (brachytherapy) [10]. About 50% of cancer patients will receive radiation therapy at some point, either as a primary treatment or adjuvant (after surgery to kill microscopic disease). Radiation is highly effective for localized tumors and is often used for cancers of the head and neck, cervix, prostate, brain, and others. Modern techniques like IMRT (intensity-modulated radiation therapy) and stereotactic radiosurgery allow very precise targeting of tumors while sparing surrounding healthy tissue. Common side effects are localized to the area treated (for example, skin irritation in the radiation field, or fatigue).
- **Chemotherapy**: Chemotherapy refers to drugs that kill rapidly dividing cells in effect, poisoning cancer cells. Unlike surgery or radiation which target a specific area, chemo is usually a systemic treatment (drugs travel through the bloodstream to reach cancer throughout the body). There are many chemotherapy agents with

different mechanisms: some directly damage DNA; others interfere with cell division or metabolism. Chemotherapy is a cornerstone for many cancers, especially those that are advanced or have spread. For instance, leukemia and lymphoma often require chemotherapy as the main treatment; cancers like breast, lung, and colon frequently use chemo either before surgery (to shrink tumors), after surgery (to eliminate stray cancer cells), or when metastasized. While chemotherapy can be very effective, it also affects some normal fast-growing cells, leading to side effects like hair loss, nausea, lowered blood counts, and risk of infections [10]. Doctors carefully balance the drug combinations and dosing to maximize cancer kill and minimize toxicity. In recent years, new formulations and supportive care (anti-nausea drugs, growth factors) have made chemo more tolerable.

- **Immunotherapy**: Immunotherapy (also called biological therapy) is a revolutionary approach that empowers the body's own immune system to fight cancer. Cancer can evade the immune system's surveillance; immunotherapy tries to remove those brakes. One form is checkpoint inhibitors, drugs that block proteins (like PD-1/PD-L1 or CTLA-4) which cancers use to turn off immune cells "releasing the brakes" so T cells can attack the tumor. This approach has led to dramatic, long-term responses in some patients with advanced melanoma, lung cancer, kidney cancer, and others. Another form is CAR-T cell therapy, where a patient's T-cells are genetically engineered to target cancer cells, effective in some leukemias and lymphomas. Immunotherapies can sometimes cause unique side effects (since revving up the immune system can lead to inflammation in the body's organs), but they have opened a new pillar of cancer treatment. In essence, immunotherapy helps the immune system "see" and attack cancer as an intruder [10]. Not all cancers respond to immunotherapy, but ongoing research is expanding its reach.
- **Targeted Therapy**: Targeted drugs are designed to specifically target molecular abnormalities in cancer cells, sparing most normal cells. For example, if cancer is driven by an overactive protein due to gene mutation, a targeted drug can block that protein. One famous example is imatinib (Gleevec) for chronic myeloid leukemia, which inhibits the BCR-ABL tyrosine kinase produced by the Philadelphia chromosome abnormality turning a once-deadly leukemia into a manageable condition. Other examples include EGFR inhibitors for lung cancers with EGFR mutations, HER2-targeted drugs (like trastuzumab) for HER2-positive breast cancer, and BRAF inhibitors for melanoma with BRAF mutations. "Targeted drug treatment focuses on specific abnormalities within cancer cells that allow them to survive." [10] Because they home in on pathways, these drugs often have different (and sometimes milder) side effect profiles compared to standard chemotherapy. However, cancers can develop resistance to targeted therapies over time by finding alternative pathways or additional mutations. Combining targeted agents with other treatments is an active area of research.
- **Hormone Therapy**: This is a subtype of targeted therapy often listed separately. Some cancers depend on hormones to grow, for instance, estrogen fuels many breast cancers, and testosterone fuels most prostate cancers. Hormone therapy uses drugs (or surgery) to reduce hormone levels or block their effect on cancer cells

[10]. Examples include tamoxifen or aromatase inhibitors for estrogen-receptor-positive breast cancer, and androgen deprivation therapy for prostate cancer. By cutting off the hormonal "fuel," these treatments can induce remission or slow cancer growth, often with relatively manageable side effects. Hormone therapies are a standard part of treatment for hormone-sensitive cancers and can be given over long periods.

- **Palliative Care**: Not a direct cancer-killing treatment, palliative care is an essential component of cancer management focused on improving quality of life. It involves relieving symptoms and side effects, and addressing the emotional, social, and spiritual needs of patients. Palliative care is appropriate at any stage of cancer, not only end-of-life. For example, pain management, treating nausea, ensuring good nutrition, and providing psychosocial support are all palliative interventions. In advanced cancer that cannot be cured, palliative treatments (like pain medication, radiation to painful metastases, or procedures to relieve obstructions) become the mainstay to help patients live as well as possible for as long as possible [11]. Importantly, palliative care works alongside curative treatments too studies show that integrating palliative care early can improve not just comfort but also sometimes survival and family well-being [12]. It is distinct from hospice care (which is focused on end-of-life); palliative care is "supportive care or symptom management" throughout the cancer journey [11].
- **Other Methods and Multimodal Therapy**: In many cases, optimal cancer treatment uses a combination of the above methods (multimodal therapy). For example, a patient with breast cancer might have surgery first, then chemotherapy, then radiation and hormonal therapy, each modality addressing a specific need (local control, systemic control, etc.). There are also emerging therapies such as gene therapy, oncolytic virus therapy (viruses that infect and kill cancer cells), and precision medicine approaches that customize treatment based on an individual's tumor genetics. Furthermore, clinical trials are continually testing new treatments; participation in trials can be an important option, especially when standard treatments are limited. Lastly, supportive care like bone marrow transplants (to rescue bone marrow after high-dose chemo) [10], or interventions like tumor treating fields (TTF) for certain brain tumors, also play roles in specific situations.

In summary, cancer treatment often involves a complex plan that may include one or several of the methods above. The overall objectives can vary, some treatments aim to cure the cancer, others aim to control it for as long as possible, and always there is an emphasis on maintaining the patient's quality of life. Thanks to decades of research, doctors today have many tools at their disposal, and treatment is usually managed by a multidisciplinary team (surgeons, medical oncologists, radiation oncologists, etc.) working together to give the patient the best outcome.

1.2 Lung Anatomy

Figure 1.1 shows the anatomy of the human respiratory system, highlighting the lungs and airways. The lungs are two sponge-like organs in the chest, responsible for gas exchange (oxygen uptake and carbon dioxide removal). Each lung is divided into lobes—the right lung has three lobes (upper, middle, lower) and the left lung has two lobes (upper and lower) [13]. The left lung is slightly smaller than the right lung because the heart occupies space on the left side of the chest [13]. The lungs are flanked by the ribs and chest wall at the sides, with the heart nestled between them in the center (mediastinum). A thin double-layered membrane called the pleura surrounds each lung. One layer of the pleura (visceral pleura) adheres to the lung surface and the other layer (parietal pleura) lines the chest wall; the pleural space between them contains a small amount of fluid that allows the lungs to glide smoothly during breathing. This setup helps prevent friction as the lungs expand and contract. Below the lungs is a large, dome-shaped muscle called the diaphragm, which separates the chest cavity from the abdominal cavity [13]. The diaphragm is the primary muscle of respiration when it contracts and moves downward, it creates suction that draws air into the lungs; when it relaxes and moves upward, it helps push air out.

The structure of the airways within the lungs resembles an upside-down tree, often called the bronchial tree. When you inhale, air enters through the nose or mouth, travels down the trachea (windpipe), and then into two main bronchi one going into each lung. The bronchi are tubular airways that further branch repeatedly inside the lungs, like branches of a tree. The first divisions form the lobar bronchi (going to each lobe), then segmental bronchi (serving regions of each lobe), and so on,

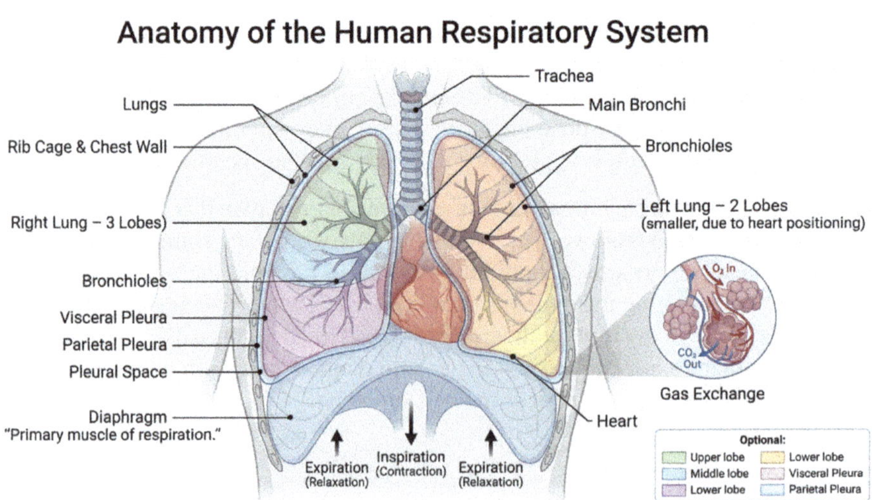

Fig. 1.1 Anatomy of the human respiratory system

becoming smaller and more numerous. The smallest conducting airways are called bronchioles, which are less than 1 mm in diameter and have no cartilage support. These bronchioles eventually lead air into clusters of microscopic air sacs called alveoli [13]. Alveoli are tiny (on the order of 0.2 mm) sac-like structures; an adult's lungs contain an estimated 300–500 million alveoli in total, creating a huge surface area for gas exchange. The alveoli are arranged in clusters (alveolar sacs) at the end of each bronchiole, rather like bunches of grapes. Each alveolus is wrapped in a fine mesh of capillaries (tiny blood vessels). Here is where the magic of respiration happens: oxygen from the air within the alveoli diffuses through the thin alveolar wall into the blood in the capillaries, and carbon dioxide from the blood diffuses into the alveoli to be exhaled. This gas exchange is the primary function of the lungs supplying oxygen to the body and eliminating the waste gas CO_2. The continuous circulation of blood through the lung capillaries and the rhythmic inflow and outflow of air (ventilation) ensure that this exchange sustains life.

The lung's architecture also includes an intricate network of blood vessels. The pulmonary arteries carry oxygen-poor blood from the heart's right ventricle into the lungs, branching alongside the bronchi, down to the capillary level around alveoli. After picking up oxygen in the alveoli, the blood is carried back to the heart's left atrium via the pulmonary veins to be pumped out to the body [14]. The lungs also have their own separate bronchial circulation (small arteries stemming from the aorta) that nourish the lung tissue itself. Additionally, lymphatic vessels in the lungs help drain excess fluid and play a role in immune defense, filtering through lymph nodes located around the bronchi (these lymph nodes are often sites where lung cancer can spread first). Structurally, the lungs are soft and elastic, which allows them to expand with each breath. The internal airspaces (alveoli) give them a spongy texture. They are relatively light (about 1 kg combined) and can float in water due to the air content.

Understanding lung anatomy is important in the context of lung cancer, because the location and spread of a tumor within these structures (lobes, bronchi, pleura, etc.) affect symptoms and treatment. For example, a tumor in a main bronchus might cause a persistent cough or wheeze and could potentially block airflow to a part of the lung, causing collapse or infection behind the blockage. A tumor on the periphery of the lung near the pleura might cause chest pain or a pleural effusion (fluid build-up) if it irritates the pleural membrane. Cancers in the upper lobes versus lower lobes might have different patterns of spread to lymph nodes. Also, since the lungs are richly supplied by blood and lymphatic vessels, lung cancers could spread (metastasize) early to other parts of the body like lymph nodes, brain, liver, and bones. All these clinical considerations are tied back to the anatomy of the lungs described above.

1.3 What is Lung Cancer?

Lung cancer is a malignant tumor that originates in the tissues of the lung, usually in the cells lining the bronchi or smaller airways. In simple terms, it is "a type of cancer that starts in the lungs" [15]. As lung cells undergo genetic mutations and begin to grow uncontrollably, they form a mass (tumor) that can interfere with lung function and eventually spread beyond the lungs. Lung cancer is not a single disease; there are several types, but they are broadly categorized into two main groups with distinct behavior and treatment approaches [15]:

- **Non-small Cell Lung Cancer (NSCLC)**: This is the more common category, accounting for about 80–85% of lung cancer cases. NSCLC encompasses multiple subtypes of lung cancers that are grouped together because their clinical management is similar [15]. The three main subtypes are:
  - **Adenocarcinoma**, the most common type of lung cancer in both smokers and non-smokers. It arises from glandular cells (for example, cells that secrete mucus) in the lung periphery [15]. Adenocarcinoma often occurs in the outer regions of the lungs and tends to grow more slowly than other types. It's also the predominant type seen in people who have never smoked.
  - **Squamous Cell Carcinoma** originates in the flat squamous cells that line the larger airways of the lungs (bronchi). It often develops in the central parts of the lung (near a main bronchus). Squamous carcinoma is strongly linked to smoking history and may be cavitated (from hollow spaces) in the lung.
  - **Large Cell Carcinoma**, an undifferentiated carcinoma that can appear in any part of the lung and tends to grow and spread quickly. This is a diagnosis of exclusion when cells don't clearly show adenocarcinoma or squamous features under the microscope. One subtype of large cell carcinoma is large-cell neuroendocrine carcinoma, which is aggressive and shares some similarities with small cell lung cancer [15].

Other less common NSCLC subtypes (like adenosquamous carcinoma or sarcomatoid carcinoma) exist but are rare. Generally, NSCLCs are relatively slower growing than small cell lung cancer, and if detected at an early stage, they can often be treated with surgery and have a chance for cure. However, NSCLCs can and do metastasize (spread) to other organs common spread sites include lymph nodes, brain, bones, liver, and adrenal glands. The prognosis varies widely by stage; early-stage NSCLC can be cured in a significant fraction of cases, while advanced metastatic NSCLC is usually not curable but may be managed for some time with systemic therapies.

- **Small Cell Lung Cancer (SCLC)**: This type comprises about 10–15% of lung cancers [15]. It is also known by older names like "oat cell carcinoma" due to the oat-grain appearance of the cells under a microscope. SCLC almost always occurs in smokers and is typically found in the central parts of the lungs (near the bronchi). Small cell lung cancer is characterized by a very rapid growth rate and a tendency to spread early and extensively to other organs [15]. Often by the time SCLC is diagnosed, it has already metastasized beyond the lungs (for example, to lymph nodes, bone marrow, liver, or brain). The aggressive nature of SCLC makes it challenging to treat surgery usually isn't an option because by diagnosis it's rarely localized enough to remove. However, SCLC tends to be initially very responsive to chemotherapy and radiation, which can cause dramatic tumor shrinkage. Unfortunately, SCLC also has a high tendency to recur (return) after initial treatment, often within months. The disease can then progress rapidly. The overall prognosis for SCLC is poor, with only a small minority of patients surviving long-term, reflecting the urgent need for new therapies. Still, it's important to note that SCLC patients can have meaningful responses to treatment that relieve symptoms and prolong life, even if cure is elusive in most cases.

Beyond these two main categories, the lungs can also be the site of rarer tumors such as carcinoid tumors (slow-growing neuroendocrine tumors, less than 5% of lung tumors [15]) or other unusual cancers like sarcomas and lymphomas that start in the lungs, but these are uncommon. When we speak of "lung cancer" in general, we are usually referring to NSCLC and SCLC. In terms of general behavior, lung cancers are particularly notorious for their lethal nature. There are a few reasons for this:

- The lungs are a vital organ, so even a local tumor can compromise breathing. Symptoms like persistent cough, coughing up blood, chest pain, or shortness of breath often don't appear until the cancer advances.
- The rich network of blood vessels and lymphatics in the lungs provides cancer cells ample routes to spread. Lung cancer frequently metastasizes the brain (which can cause headaches, seizures), bones (causing pain or fractures), liver, and adrenal glands, among other sites.
- Many lung cancers are linked to smoking, which may have caused damage throughout the respiratory tract, so patients might also have other lung issues (like COPD) that complicate treatment.
- Historically, there were limited effective treatments for advanced lung cancer. However, this has been changing recently, especially for certain subsets of NSCLC where targeted therapies and immunotherapies have significantly improved outcomes.

It's sobering that lung cancer remains the leading cause of cancer death worldwide, accounting for about 18% of all cancer deaths [1, 9]. In 2022, lung cancer caused an estimated 1.8 million deaths globally, more than the next two deadliest cancers (colorectal and liver) combined [9]. Part of this high toll is due to how common lung cancer is (it's one of the top diagnosed cancers), but part is also due to its aggressive nature and the fact that it is often diagnosed at a late stage when cure is difficult. The five-year survival rate for lung cancer in many countries is on order of 20% or less, though it varies by stage (with early-stage NSCLC having much better outlook than extensive SCLC, for example).

In summary, lung cancer is a malignant disease of the lung's cells, most often caused by tobacco smoke exposure, and it comes in two primary forms with distinct profiles. NSCLC is more common and sometimes curable if caught early; SCLC is less common but very aggressive. Both types can cause serious illness by invading lung structures and spreading to distant organs. In the following sections, we will delve into the specific risk factors for lung cancer and approaches to prevention, which are crucial given the magnitude of this disease.

1.4 Risk Factors for Lung Cancer

Lung cancer has well-established risk factors, the most prominent of which is tobacco smoking. However, there are several other factors from environmental exposures to genetic susceptibility that also contribute to lung cancer risk. Key risk factors include:

- **Cigarette Smoking**: Smoking is by far the first risk factor for lung cancer. Roughly 85% of all lung cancer cases are attributable to tobacco use [9]. Smokers have dramatically higher lung cancer rates than never-smokers, and heavy smokers (in terms of cigarettes per day and years of use) are at the highest risk. Inhaled tobacco smoke delivers a cocktail of carcinogens (such as benzo[a]pyrene and nitrosamines) that cause DNA mutations in lung cells. Over time, this can initiate cancer development. Smoking also harms the lung's clearance mechanisms (like the cilia), making it harder to eliminate toxins. It's important to note that secondhand smoke (breathing other people's tobacco smoke) also increases lung cancer risk in never-smokers [9]. There is no safe level of smoking even "light" or occasional smoking and exposure to secondhand smoke carry risk. Cigar and pipe smoking, while somewhat different in inhalation patterns, are also linked to lung cancer (though the risk is somewhat lower than cigarettes). The good news is that quitting smoking at any age significantly reduces risk over time (see Sect. 1.5 on Prevention). Populations that have reduced smoking have seen proportional drops in lung cancer incidence, reinforcing this causal link [1].
- **Radon Exposure**: Radon is a radioactive gas that emerges naturally from soil and rocks. It can accumulate in enclosed spaces like homes (especially basements). Radon is the second leading cause of lung cancer after smoking, and the leading cause among non-smokers [16]. Radon decays into radioactive particles that, when inhaled, can damage lung cell DNA. The risk from radon is compounded for smokers (smoking + radon exposure has a supra-additive effect on lung cancer risk) [17]. Radon-related lung cancers are estimated to account for about 20,000 deaths per year in the U.S. [16]. Testing homes for radon and remediating high levels (through ventilation systems, for instance) is an important prevention strategy, particularly in areas known to have high radon levels.
- **Occupational and Environmental Carcinogens**: Certain substances encountered in the workplace or environment can cause lung cancer. One of the most notorious is asbestos, a fibrous material once used extensively in construction and industry. Asbestos exposure increases the risk of lung cancer significantly, especially in smokers (the combination is particularly deadly) [3]. It also causes

mesothelioma, a different cancer of the pleura. Other occupational lung carcinogens include silica dust (miners, sandblasting, masonry can be exposed silica can cause lung scarring and cancer) [3], diesel exhaust (people who work around heavy diesel machinery or truck drivers breathing fumes have a higher risk) [3], certain metallic dusts (like arsenic, chromium, nickel in industrial settings), coal smoke and soot (historically seen in chimney sweeps as Pott observed, and indoor coal burning for heating can increase risk), and ionizing radiation (apart from radon, medical or nuclear industry exposures). Even occupations like painters (exposed to solvent fumes) or rubber manufacturers have been noted to have elevated lung cancer rates in some studies. Environmental air pollution in urban areas (from vehicles, power plants, etc.) also contributes long-term exposure to fine particulate matter (PM2.5) and other pollutants have been classified as a cause of lung cancer by the WHO. In the UK, for example, it's estimated that about 8% of lung cancer cases are due to outdoor air pollution [3]. While individual risk from pollution is small compared to smoking, widespread exposure makes it a significant public health factor.

- **Personal or Family History and Genetics**: A family history of lung cancer (having a close relative with lung cancer) modestly increases one's risk of developing lung cancer [3]. This could be due to shared genetic factors, shared environmental exposures (like a smoking household), or both. Some people may inherit genetic traits that make them more susceptible to the harmful effects of tobacco or slower detoxify carcinogens. Additionally, certain rare inherited syndromes (e.g., Li-Fraumeni syndrome caused by TP53 gene mutations, or EGFR mutations in some East Asian families) can predispose individuals to lung cancer even without smoking. However, there is no single "lung cancer gene" that guarantees the disease genetics likely influence risk in a polygenic way (multiple genes each conferring a small increase in risk). For smokers, having a family history might elevate risk beyond the very high baseline risk that smoking confers (some studies suggest smokers with a family history are at even higher risk than smokers without such history). Nonetheless, avoiding smoking greatly attenuates any genetic predisposition's impact. It's also worth noting that people who have had one lung cancer are at risk of developing a second lung cancer, especially if they continue to smoke, because the entire respiratory epithelium has been exposed to carcinogens.
- **Previous Lung Diseases**: Lung diseases that cause chronic inflammation or scaring can increase lung cancer risk. For instance, Chronic Obstructive Pulmonary Disease (COPD) and pulmonary fibrosis are associated with higher lung cancer rates, independent of smoking (though smoking often underlies those diseases as well) [3]. Prior tuberculosis infection leaves scarred areas in the lung that can be sites for a type of cancer called scar carcinoma. While these conditions are not primary causes like smoking, they can contribute to risk and make diagnosis tricky (a new cancer might be initially mistaken for a flare of an old disease).

In summary, the risk factors for lung cancer are led by smoking (active and passive), a truly dominant factor followed by other inhaled carcinogens like radon, asbestos, and pollution, plus genetic and medical factors. Importantly, many of these risk factors are preventable or avoidable. That is why public health efforts focus heavily on tobacco control (prevention and cessation), radon abatement, reducing occupational exposures, and improving air quality. These efforts have started to pay off lung cancer rates have plateaued or declined in some countries as smoking prevalence has dropped and workplace hazards have been mitigated [1]. Still, lung cancer remains all too common, and understanding its risk factors helps identify who should be screened and what interventions can save lives.

1.5 Prevention Against Lung Cancer

Preventing lung cancer (or any cancer) involves reducing exposure to known risk factors and taking proactive measures to detect disease early. Given lung cancer's strong link to modifiable behaviors and environmental exposures, effective prevention could dramatically reduce its incidence and mortality. Here are the main strategies for lung cancer prevention and early detection:

- **Smoking Cessation and Tobacco Control**: The most powerful preventive measure against lung cancer is to never smoke, or if one is a smoker, to quit smoking. Quitting smoking at any age significantly lowers the risk of developing lung cancer. In fact, about 10 years after quitting, a former smoker's risk of lung cancer drops to roughly half the risk of someone who continues to smoke [18]. The longer one remains smoke-free, the more the risk continues to decline, although it may never quite return to the baseline of a never-smoker. For example, after 15–20 years of cessation, the risk can approach that of a non-smoker, depending on how much one smoked before [18, 19]. On a public health level, countries have implemented various tobacco control policies: higher taxes on cigarettes, bans on advertising, graphic warning labels, smoke-free public spaces, and plain packaging. These measures have proven effective in reducing smoking rates and hence future lung cancer cases. Additionally, preventing the initiation of smoking (especially in youth) is critical. Education campaigns and smoking cessation programs (nicotine replacement therapy, medications like varenicline, counseling, quitlines) are all part of comprehensive tobacco control. The impact of these efforts is evident in statistics for instance; lung cancer rates have been falling among men in many countries in line with dropping smoking rates decades earlier [1]. Avoidance of other forms of tobacco (cigars, pipes, chewing tobacco) and of secondhand smoke also falls under this umbrella. Even exposure to smoke residues (thirdhand smoke) is being studied for potential harm. In summary, "it's never too late to quit" and never too early to prevent the habit from forming.

- **Reduction of Occupational and Environmental Exposures**: Another pillar of lung cancer prevention is minimizing inhalation of known carcinogens aside from tobacco. For radon, this means testing homes (especially in high-risk geographic areas) and fixing any high levels (for example, improving under-house ventilation or sealing cracks in foundations). Public health agencies provide guidelines for safe radon levels and often offer radon testing kits to homeowners. For occupational carcinogens like asbestos, silica, coal dust, arsenic, and diesel exhaust, regulatory standards and workplace protections are key. This includes wearing appropriate respiratory protective equipment, using proper ventilation systems in mines or factories, substituting safer materials when possible, and following exposure limit guidelines. Many countries have banned or strictly limited asbestos use (as noted, the UK banned asbestos in 1999 [3], and other countries have similar regulations). Workers who are at risk (e.g., miners, construction workers, industrial workers) often undergo periodic health screenings, including lung function tests and imaging, to catch any early changes. For air pollution, prevention is more complex as it requires broader policy transitioning to cleaner energy, reducing vehicle emissions, and urban planning to improve air quality. Individuals can partly protect themselves by avoiding heavy outdoor exertion on days with poor air quality or using air purifiers indoors, but the larger solution is societal. All these measures contribute to a lower burden of carcinogens that can trigger lung cancer.
- **Diet and General Health**: While not as potent as smoking cessation, maintaining a healthy lifestyle supports lung health. Some studies suggest that diets rich in fruits and vegetables (which contain antioxidants) might help protect against lung cancer, especially for smokers or former smokers but the evidence is mixed. What's clear is that taking high-dose beta-carotene supplements as a smoker is harmful: trials found that heavy smokers who took beta-carotene had increased lung cancer rates [3], so supplements are not a shortcut to prevention and can be dangerous in that context. A balanced diet and regular exercise contribute to overall health and may help the body fend off diseases in general. Keeping the immune system strong (e.g., avoiding chronic inflammatory states, treating infections promptly) could be beneficial since chronic lung infections or inflammation can elevate cancer risk. Preventive healthcare like getting the flu vaccine or pneumonia vaccine can also indirectly help by maintaining better lung function and less lung damage over time.
- **Screening and Early Detection**: Prevention isn't only about stopping cancer from occurring; it's also about catching it early when it's most treatable (which is sometimes called secondary prevention). For lung cancer, early detection through screening has become a recommended strategy for high-risk populations. Specifically, annual low-dose CT (LDCT) scans of the chest can find lung cancers at an earlier, curable stage in people at elevated risk. Based on evidence from large trials, organizations like the American Cancer Society and the U.S. Preventive Services Task Force now recommend yearly LDCT screening for adults roughly age 50 to 80 who have a significant smoking history (usually defined as at least a 20 pack-year history) and who currently smoke or quit within the past 15 years [20,

21]. Screening is not for everyone—it has potential downsides like false positives or finding benign nodules that require follow-up—but for the high-risk group, benefits outweigh risks. Research shows that screening can reduce lung cancer mortality by about 20% in those high-risk individuals [22], by detecting tumors when they are small and before symptoms appear. Early-stage lung cancers found on screening can often be surgically removed or treated with curative intent, dramatically improving survival odds. Aside from formal screening programs, raising awareness about lung cancer symptoms among clinicians and the public is important: if a person (especially a smoker) has a persistent cough, coughing blood, or unexplained weight loss, prompt evaluation (even if they feel otherwise okay) can lead to earlier diagnosis.

- **Policy Measures and Societal Efforts**: On a broader scale, lung cancer prevention is bolstered by legislative and policy efforts. Examples include laws banning smoking in workplaces, restaurants, and bars (protecting people from secondhand smoke and also creating an environment that encourages smokers to quit), tobacco taxation (one of the most effective means to reduce tobacco use, especially among price-sensitive groups like youth), plain packaging and graphic warnings on cigarette packs, and public education campaigns (like mass media anti-tobacco ads). Some countries have run successful anti-smoking campaigns that significantly cut smoking rates. Healthcare systems also have a role: ensuring that every patient who smokes is advised to quit and offered help is a form of preventive care. Environmental policies that target air quality (such as emissions standards for factories and vehicles) contribute to lowering lung cancer risk in the population over time. Furthermore, occupational safety agencies enforcing exposure limits and proper protective equipment in industries help prevent future cases of occupational lung cancer.
- **Chemoprevention and Vaccines**: Unlike some other cancers (such as cervical cancer, which can be prevented by an HPV vaccine), there is no vaccine to prevent lung cancer. However, vaccines that prevent infections like Flu or COVID-19 indirectly help lung health. Still there are ways to develop vaccine using in silico methods or reverse vaccinology using immunoinformatic approach for cancer prevention [23, 24]. Researchers have explored chemoprevention medications or supplements to reduce lung cancer risk (for instance, trials of vitamin A derivatives in smokers) but so far, no drug has shown a clear benefit for lung cancer prevention in smokers without doing harm. The best "medicine" remains quitting smoking. For certain occupational risks, sometimes prophylactic measures are taken (like administering inhaled corticosteroids to reduce inflammation in high-risk miners, though this is not standard for cancer prevention).

In conclusion, lung cancer is largely a preventable tragedy. Our earlier studies have predicted the onset of lung cancer using machine learning approach [25]. Public health experts often note that if nobody smoked, lung cancer would become a rare disease. Of course, not all lung cancers would vanish (non-smoker cases exist due to radon, genetics, etc.), but the incidence would be a fraction of what it is today. Thus, prevention efforts focus heavily on tobacco control, but also on clean air and safe workplaces, and on screening those at highest risk to catch cancer early. A multi-faceted approach involving individuals (making healthy choices), healthcare providers (supporting prevention and early detection), and policymakers (enacting health-protective laws) offers the best chance to reduce the burden of lung cancer in the coming decades. Every percentage point drop-in smoking rate and every high-risk individual screened contributes to lives saved, as evidenced by the statistics and research we have done so far. Through such continued efforts, there is hope that lung cancer will claim far fewer lives in future than it does today [1, 22].

1.6 Summary

This chapter provides a comprehensive overview of lung cancer, its causes, classification, diagnosis, and treatment methods, along with strategies for prevention. Cancer is a group of diseases characterized by uncontrolled cell growth and is a leading global cause of death. Lung cancer, primarily caused by smoking, is the most lethal cancer worldwide, with two main types: non-small cell lung cancer (NSCLC) and small cell lung cancer (SCLC). NSCLC is more common and has a better prognosis if detected early, while SCLC is aggressive and often diagnosed at advanced stages. Risk factors for lung cancer include smoking, radon exposure, occupational and environmental carcinogens, genetic predisposition, and previous lung diseases. Effective prevention strategies include smoking cessation, reducing exposure to carcinogens, maintaining a healthy lifestyle, and implementing screening programs for high-risk individuals. Diagnosis involves imaging tests, biopsies, tumor markers, and molecular testing, while treatment options include surgery, radiation, chemotherapy, immunotherapy, targeted therapy, and palliative care. The chapter emphasizes the importance of public health efforts, policy measures, and early detection in reducing the global burden of lung cancer.

References

1. Nwosu, N. (2024). Cancer: A disease of modern times? *Cureus, 16*(11).
2. Latest global cancer data: Cancer burden rises to 19.3 million new cases and 10.0 million cancer deaths in 2020. Weblink: https://www.iarc.who.int/news-events/latest-global-cancer-data-cancer-burden-rises-to-19-3-million-new-cases-and-10-0-million-cancer-deaths-in-2020/#:~:text=The%20global%20cancer%20burden%20is,women%20die%20from%20the%20disease. Last Access: January 2026.
3. Risks and causes of lung cancer. Website: https://www.cancerresearchuk.org/about-cancer/lung-cancer/risks-causes. Last Access: January 2026.
4. Milestones in cancer research and discovery. Website: https://www.cancer.gov/research/progress/250-years-milestones. Last Access: January 2026.
5. Laguna, J. C., Moreno, L., Potrony, M., Grau, E., Pastor, B., Mena-Guerrero, J., Jiménez, M., Gorria, T., Puig-Butillé, J. A., Reguart, N., Cajal, T. R.,Teixido, C., & Mezquita, L. (2025).

Prevalence and characteristics of lung cancer in families harboring Pathogenic Germline Variants in cancer predisposing genes: A 20-year retrospective analysis. *European Journal of Cancer*, *225*, 115571.

6. Cancer classification. Website: https://training.seer.cancer.gov/disease/categories/classification.html. Last Access: January 2026.
7. Mandal, A. Cancer classification. Website: https://www.news-medical.net/health/Cancer-Classification.aspx. Last Access: January 2026.
8. Carbone, A. (2020). Cancer classification at the crossroads. *Cancers, 12*(4), 980.
9. Lung cancer. Website: https://www.iarc.who.int/cancer-type/lung-cancer/. Last Access: January 2026.
10. Cancer—Diagnosis and treatment. Website: https://www.mayoclinic.org/diseases-conditions/cancer/diagnosis-treatment/drc-20370594. Last Access: January 2026.
11. Palliative care. Website: https://www.cancer.org/cancer/supportive-care/palliative-care.html. Last Access: January 2026.
12. Meier, D. E., & Brawley, O. W. (2011). Palliative care and the quality of life. *Journal of Clinical Oncology, 29*(20), 2750.
13. Respiratory system. Website: https://www.cancer.org/cancer/understanding-cancer/anatomy-gallery/respiratory-system.html. Last Access: January 2026.
14. Lung. Website: https://en.wikipedia.org/wiki/Lung. Last Access: January 2026.
15. What is lung cancer? Website: https://www.cancer.org/cancer/types/lung-cancer/about/what-is.html. Last Access: January 2026.
16. Radon and cancer risk. Website: https://www.cancer.org/cancer/risk-prevention/radiation-exposure/radon.html. Last Access: January 2026.
17. Radon is the Nation's 2nd leading cause of lung cancer. Website: https://www.lung.org/media/press-releases/fy25-radon-action-month-release. Last Access: January 2026.
18. Health benefits of quitting smoking over time. Website: https://www.cancer.org/cancer/risk-prevention/tobacco/guide-quitting-smoking/benefits-of-quitting-smoking-over-time.html. Last Access: January 2026.
19. Smoking and cancer. Website: https://www.cdc.gov/tobacco/campaign/tips/diseases/cancer.html. Last Access: January 2026.
20. Lung cancer: Screening. Website: https://www.uspreventiveservicestaskforce.org/uspstf/recommendation/lung-cancer-screening. Last Access: January 2026.
21. Lung cancer screening guidelines. Website: https://www.cancer.org/health-care-professionals/american-cancer-society-prevention-early-detection-guidelines/lung-cancer-screening-guidelines.html. Last Access: January 2026.
22. Lung cancer key findings. Website: https://www.lung.org/research/state-of-lung-cancer/key-findings. Last Access: January 2026.
23. Mathur, N., Sai Chandragiri, S., Sarita, Shandily, S., Mukeshbhai Santoki, K., Navinchandra Vadhavana, N., Shah, S., & Chandra, M. (2024). In silico docking: Protocols for computational exploration of molecular interactions. In *Biomedical engineering*. IntechOpen. https://doi.org/10.5772/intechopen.1005527
24. Manvani, R., Purohit, H., Sahoo, C. R., Rajput, M., & Shah, S. (2024). Chapter 5—Immunoinformatics: An interdisciplinary technique for designing and engineering vaccine antigen. In J. Das, S. Dave, S. de Castro Soares, S. Tiwari (Eds.), *Reverse vaccinology* (pp. 87–99). Academic Press. ISBN 9780443133954. https://doi.org/10.1016/B978-0-443-13395-4.00012-5
25. Trivedi, D., Munshi, S., Diwan, A., & Shah, S. (2023). Enhancing lung cancer prediction through machine learning: A data-driven approach. In *2023 IEEE 11th region 10 humanitarian technology conference (R10-HTC)*, Rajkot, India, pp. 1150–1155. https://doi.org/10.1109/R10-HTC57504.2023.10461923

Chapter 2
Types, Diagnosis, and Treatment of Lung Cancer

Lung cancer is among the most common cancers and is the leading cause of cancer death worldwide [1]. It generally refers to malignancies that originate in the lung tissues (usually the bronchi, bronchioles, or alveoli) as opposed to cancers that spread to the lungs from elsewhere. Lung cancer is often diagnosed at advanced stages due to its tendency to cause symptoms only in later stages, which contributes to its high mortality. However, advances in early detection (such as screening with low-dose CT scans) and new treatments (like targeted drugs and immunotherapies) are improving outcomes. This chapter will discuss the types of lung cancer, how it is staged and diagnosed (including early detection methods), and the range of treatments available for lung cancer.

2.1 Stages of Lung Cancer

Lung cancer staging describes how far the cancer has progressed, which is crucial for guiding treatment and estimating prognosis. The staging system most used is the AJCC (American Joint Committee on Cancer) TNM system, which assigns [2]:

- T (Tumor): the size/extent of the primary tumor in the lung;
- N (Nodes): whether cancer has spread to nearby lymph nodes;
- M (Metastasis): whether it has spread to distant organs.

Various combinations of T, N, and M values are then grouped into an overall stage (0, I, II, III, or IV) [2]. In broad terms, lower stage numbers indicate more limited cancer, while higher stages (like Stage IV) indicate more extensive spread. Staging may be assessed clinically (based on imaging tests and biopsies) and then confirmed pathologically if surgery is done (by examining resected tissue) [2]. Below is an overview of lung cancer stages:

S. Shah and R. Thanki, *Artificial Intelligence for Early Detection and Diagnosis of Lung Cancer*, Signals and Communication Technology,
https://doi.org/10.1007/978-3-032-29615-3_2

2.1.1 Stage 0

Stage 0 lung cancer (carcinoma in situ) is the earliest stage. The cancer is found only in the top layer of cells lining an airway and has not invaded deeper lung tissues or spread to lymph nodes or other organs [2, 3]. In this stage, the tumor is essentially non-invasive. Stage 0 is uncommon in lung cancer, but when it occurs, it is highly curable, often managed with surgical removal of the abnormal cells before they turn into an invasive cancer. There is no spread to lymph nodes (N0) and no metastasis (M0) by definition [2].

2.1.2 Stage I and Stage II

Stage I lung cancer is an early, localized cancer. The tumor is confined to the lung and has not spread to any lymph nodes or distant sites [4]. Typically, Stage I tumors are smaller in size. In TNM terms, this corresponds to T1 or T2 tumors with N0, M0. Patients with Stage I disease often have no or minimal symptoms, and cancer may be discovered incidentally or via screening.

Stage II lung cancer is a locally advanced stage compared to I. Stage II tumors are either larger in size or have spread to nearby lymph nodes inside the lung, or there may be multiple tumor nodules in the same lobe of the lung [4]. For example, Stage IIA/B might involve a tumor that is growing larger than Stage I or has invaded nearby structures, and/or it has reached the hilar or intrapulmonary lymph nodes on the same side, but no distant spread has occurred [3]. In summary, Stage II indicates the cancer is still limited to the chest (no distant metastasis) but with greater local extent than Stage I, either a bigger tumor, involvement of local lymph nodes, or additional tumor nodules in the same lung lobe [4]. Stages I and II are often considered "early-stage" lung cancers, for which surgery (with curative intent) is usually the primary treatment (see Sect. 2.5.1).

2.1.3 Stage III

Stage III lung cancer is considered locally advanced disease. By Stage III, the cancer has spread further regionally, this can mean it has spread to lymph nodes in the mediastinum (the center of the chest between the lungs) or to other nearby organs/ structures in the chest [3]. Stage III is often subdivided into IIIA, IIIB, and IIIC, depending on the extent:

- In Stage IIIA, the tumor might still be confined to one side of the chest but involves mediastinal lymph nodes on the same side or has grown into nearby structures.

- In Stage IIIB/IIIC, cancer may have spread to lymph nodes on the opposite side of the chest, above the collarbone, or there are multiple tumor locations in different lobes of the same lung [4].

Stage III tumors are usually too extensive to be cured by surgery alone (especially IIIB/C) and often require a combination of treatments (e.g., chemotherapy and radiation, sometimes with surgery in select IIIA cases). There is no distant organ metastasis in Stage III (M0 by definition), but the regional spread is significant. Stage III represents a critical intermediate stage: more advanced than purely local disease, but potentially still within a curative range with aggressive therapy.

2.1.4 Stage IV

Stage IV is the most advanced stage of lung cancer. In Stage IV, cancer has metastasized to distant sites beyond the original lung. This means cancer cells have traveled through the bloodstream or lymphatic system to seed new tumors in other parts of the body. Common sites of distant metastases for lung cancer include the other lungs, the pleura (lining around the lungs), the pericardium (lining around the heart), brain, bones, liver, or adrenal glands [4]. Even the presence of malignant fluid collections such as a malignant pleural effusion (fluid around the lung) or malignant pericardial effusion (fluid around the heart) classifies the disease as Stage IV, because these usually signify disseminated cancer cells [4]. Stage IV can be further split (IVA vs. IVB) depending on the number and location of metastases (for instance, a single distant metastasis might be IVA, while multiple organ metastases or spread to the other lung is IVB).

Stage IV lung cancer is generally not curable with current therapies, but it is treatable. The focus is on systemic treatments (like chemotherapy, targeted therapy, immunotherapy) to control disease, relieve symptoms, and prolong survival. Outcomes for Stage IV are much poorer than for earlier stages for example, five-year survival for distant metastatic lung cancer is only around 12%, compared to approximately 67% for localized (Stage I) disease [5]. This stark difference underscores the importance of early detection.

2.2 Types of Lung Cancer

Lung cancer is broadly categorized into two main types based on the appearance of the cancer cells under a microscope and their clinical behavior: non-small cell lung cancer (NSCLC) and small cell lung cancer (SCLC) [6]. These two categories together account for many lung cancers. They differ in how they grow, spread, and are treated.

- **Non-small Cell Lung Cancer (NSCLC)**: This is the most common type, accounting for about 80–85% of all lung cancer cases [6]. NSCLC is an umbrella term that includes several subtypes, the main ones being:
  - **Adenocarcinoma**: Arises from mucus-producing glandular cells in the lung. Adenocarcinoma is the most common subtype of NSCLC and often occurs in the outer parts of the lungs. It is the predominant type seen in non-smokers and is more common in women than men [6].
  - **Squamous Cell Carcinoma**: Originates in the squamous cells lining the bronchial tubes. It is strongly linked to smoking history and often found in central parts of the lungs near major airways [6].
  - **Large Cell Carcinoma**: A less differentiated form that can appear in any part of the lung and tends to grow and spread rapidly [6]. (There is also a variant called large cell neuroendocrine carcinoma, which is aggressive and shares some features with SCLC.)

  These subtypes are grouped as NSCLC because their treatment approaches and prognoses are similar [6]. NSCLC tends to grow and spread a bit slower than small cell cancer. If diagnosed at an early stage, NSCLC may be curable with surgery or localized therapy.
- **Small Cell Lung Cancer (SCLC)**: This type makes up about 10–15% of lung cancers [6]. SCLC is also known as "oat cell carcinoma" for the way the cells look. It is strongly associated with smoking and is characterized by a very rapid growth rate. SCLC often spreads quickly; in fact, most patients have cancer that has already spread beyond the lung at diagnosis [6]. Because of this aggressive behavior, SCLC is typically not managed with surgery (except in rare very early cases) instead, it is usually treated with chemotherapy and radiation, as it tends to respond well to these initially [6]. Unfortunately, SCLC also tends to relapse. SCLC is sometimes staged differently from NSCLC. In addition to formal TNM staging, doctors often use a simpler two-stage system for SCLC:
  - **Limited Stage**: the cancer is confined to one side of the chest (one lung and possibly nearby lymph nodes) and could be encompassed within a single radiation therapy field [4]. This roughly corresponds to earlier SCLC that is localized to the thorax.
  - **Extensive Stage**: cancer has spread more widely in the chest or to distant organs (beyond what a single radiation field could cover) [4]. Most SCLC cases are extensive at stage at diagnosis.

It's worth noting there are a few other rare types of tumors in the lung, such as lung carcinoid tumors (neuroendocrine tumors), and cancers metastatic to the lung from other sites, but these are relatively uncommon and are managed differently [6]. The discussion in this chapter will focus on primary lung cancers (NSCLC and SCLC), as they represent many cases.

2.3 Early Detection of Lung Cancer

Early detection of lung cancer greatly improves the chances of successful treatment. As mentioned, lung cancer is often asymptomatic in its initial stages, so it frequently goes undiagnosed until it has advanced. Detecting lung cancer before it spreads (while it is still in a localized Stage I or II) dramatically boosts survival odds for example, the 5-year survival rate is on the order of 60–70% when the cancer is localized to the lung, versus barely above 10% once it has metastasized to distant organs [5]. This section covers how lung cancer can be detected early, focusing on imaging and biopsy techniques. Ultimately, a biopsy (tissue sample) is required to confirm a lung cancer diagnosis, but imaging tools are critical to find suspicious nodules or masses in the first place.

2.3.1 Biopsies

A biopsy is the removal of a small sample of tissue (or cells) for examination under a microscope to determine if cancer is present. In the context of lung cancer, if an imaging scan finds a suspicious nodule or mass, a biopsy is typically performed to confirm whether it is malignant and to identify the cancer type. Only by examining cells from the lung can doctors make an actual diagnosis of lung cancer [28]. Biopsies are thus an essential component of early detection and diagnosis—an imaging test might suggest cancer, but the biopsy proves it. There are several procedures available to obtain lung tissue:

- **Needle Biopsy (Percutaneous Biopsy)**: A needle is inserted through the chest wall (skin) into the lung lesion to withdraw cells or a core of tissue [7]. This is often done under imaging guidance (such as a CT scan) to precisely target the nodule. Needle biopsies are minimally invasive (no surgical incision needed) and useful for lesions near the outer parts of the lungs. A fine needle aspiration (FNA) uses a very thin needle to suck out cells, while a core needle biopsy uses a slightly larger needle to get a tissue core [7]. The main risk is a collapsed lung (pneumothorax) if air leaks, but this is usually manageable.
- **Bronchoscopy**: A flexible camera (bronchoscope) is inserted through the airways (trachea and bronchi) to visually examine the inside of the lung passages. Through the bronchoscope, instruments can take biopsies of tumors in the central airways or sample lymph nodes via techniques like endobronchial ultrasound (EBUS) guided needle aspiration [4]. Bronchoscopy is especially useful for centrally located tumors or lymph node biopsies.
- **Endobronchial or Endoscopic Ultrasound (EBUS/EUS)**: These are specialized forms of bronchoscopy or upper endoscopy with ultrasound guidance to biopsy lymph nodes that lie just outside the airways (in the mediastinum or around

bronchi) without open surgery. An EBUS-TBNA (transbronchial needle aspiration) can sample mediastinal lymph nodes through the airway wall [3], which is extremely useful for staging (see Sect. 2.4.2).
- **Surgical Biopsies**: If less invasive methods are not diagnostic, surgery may be done to obtain tissue. Techniques include thoracoscopy or VATS (video-assisted thoracic surgery) inserting a scope and instruments through small chest incisions to access and biopsy peripheral lung lesions or pleural areas [4]. In some cases, a more extensive surgery (thoracotomy) might be needed to remove a suspicious nodule for diagnosis.
- **Thoracentesis**: This is a procedure to remove fluid from the pleural space (around the lungs) if a pleural effusion is present. If lung cancer has caused a malignant pleural effusion, cancer cells might be found in the fluid, confirming the diagnosis [7].

Importantly, when a biopsy confirms lung cancer, the tissue can also be tested for molecular markers for instance, genetic mutations or protein markers that can guide the use of targeted therapies (see Sect. 2.5.4). Common genetic alterations tested in NSCLC include EGFR, ALK, KRAS, ROS1, BRAF, MET, RET, and others [4], because specific drugs can target some of these mutations. In summary, biopsy procedures are the gateway to both confirming early lung cancers and enabling personalized treatment by tissue analysis.

2.3.2 Imaging

Imaging tests are the primary tools for detecting lung abnormalities that might be cancer. A variety of imaging modalities can visualize the lungs:

- **Chest X-Ray**: Often the first-line imaging for respiratory symptoms. A chest radiograph can sometimes reveal a lung tumor or abnormal mass. However, small early-stage lung cancers are easily missed on a plain X-ray. Studies have shown that routine chest x-rays are not effective as a screening tool to reduce lung cancer mortality [8]. So, while an X-ray is a quick initial test (for example, to investigate a persistent cough), a normal chest X-ray does not rule out lung cancer if suspicion is high. Any suspicious finding on X-ray warrants further imaging with CT.
- **Computed Tomography (CT) Scan**: CT scans are far more sensitive and detailed than X-rays. A CT scan of the chest can detect nodules just a few millimeters in size and provides a cross-sectional view of the lungs. CT is much more likely to find a lung tumor than a routine X-ray, and it can show the exact size, shape, and position of any tumor [7]. It also helps in assessing lymph node enlargement and whether the cancer might have invaded nearby structures. For these reasons, CT scanning is the cornerstone of lung cancer imaging. When lung cancer is suspected or needs to be staged, a CT of the chest (often extending through the upper abdomen to check liver/adrenals) is typically performed. CT scans can also be used to guide needle biopsies to sample deep lung lesions [7].

- **Low-Dose CT (LDCT) for Screening**: A special application of CT is low-dose CT screening in high-risk asymptomatic individuals (discussed more in Sect. 2.4.1). LDCT uses a lower radiation dose and is done routinely (annually) to look for early lung nodules before symptoms develop [8]. It has been proven to detect cancers at a smaller size/stage and to reduce lung cancer mortality in high-risk groups.
- **Magnetic Resonance Imaging (MRI)**: MRI uses magnetic fields rather than X-rays. MRI is not routine for diagnosing a lung primary tumor, but it is very useful to evaluate possible spread to certain areas, especially the brain or spinal cord. For instance, if a patient is diagnosed with lung cancer, an MRI of the brain might be done to look for any metastatic tumors (since lung cancer commonly spreads to the brain) [7]. MRI can also help clarify involvement of the chest wall or spinal column if a tumor is at the apex of the lung (as in a Pancoast tumor).
- **Positron Emission Tomography (PET) Scan**: PET is a functional imaging that highlights areas of high metabolic activity. Patients are injected with a radioactive glucose tracer (FDG); cancer cells, which consume a lot of sugar, light up on the scan. A PET scan, especially when combined with CT (PET/CT), is extremely valuable in lung cancer staging [7]. It can detect active cancer in lymph nodes or distant organs that might not be obvious on CT alone. PET/CT is now a standard part of evaluating lung cancer spread (except in the brain, where MRI is preferred, as the brain is not well-assessed by PET) [7]. If a lung nodule is found, a PET scan can also help determine if it is likely cancerous (malignant nodules usually show high uptake). PET findings often guide where to biopsy (e.g., hypermetabolic lymph nodes).
- **Bone Scan**: This is an older nuclear medicine test (now largely supplemented by PET or by specific MRI/CT when needed) that can show cancer spread to bones. A small amount of radioactive material is used to reveal "hot spots" in bone. It might be used if PET is not available and bone metastasis is suspected [7].

In the context of early detection, imaging finds the targets that need biopsy. For example, a screening low-dose CT might find an 8-mm nodule in the lung that wasn't causing any symptoms. That nodule can then be monitored or biopsied early. Imaging is also repeated during follow-up to monitor for recurrence or to assess if treatment is working (tumor shrinkage). In summary, advanced imaging modalities are indispensable in catching lung cancer early and in guiding the diagnostic and staging process.

2.4 Diagnosis of Lung Cancer

The diagnosis of lung cancer is a multistep process that usually begins with suspicion (based on symptoms or an abnormal screening test) and ends with confirming cancer and determining its extent (stage). Key elements of diagnosing lung cancer include screening high-risk people, performing diagnostic imaging and biopsies for those with suspicious findings, and staging the cancer to guide therapy. By the time a diagnosis is made, doctors will also classify the cancer type (NSCLC versus SCLC and subtype) through pathology. This section highlights the formal screening recommendations for lung cancer and how staging is performed as part of the diagnostic work-up.

2.4.1 *Screening*

Lung cancer screening refers to testing people who do not have symptoms to detect lung cancer at an early, more treatable stage. Decades of smoking history are the biggest risk factor for lung cancer, so screening programs focus on smokers and former smokers at high risk. Based on the latest guidelines, annual screening with low-dose CT (LDCT) is recommended for certain high-risk individuals. The American Cancer Society (and US Preventive Services Task Force) recommends yearly LDCT scans for adults roughly age 50–80 who have a significant smoking history (at least a 20 pack-year smoking history) and currently smoke or have quit within the past 15 years [8, 9]. (A "pack-year" means 1 pack of cigarettes per day for a year; 20 pack-years could be 1 pack a day for 20 years, or 2 packs a day for 10 years, etc. [8].)

Screening is only advised for people healthy enough to undergo potential lung cancer treatment and who are still within the age/risk window for example, if someone had serious illnesses that would prevent lung surgery or has not smoked in over 15 years, screening may not be appropriate [8]. The reason is that screening has potential downsides and it is only beneficial if the person could benefit from early cancer detection.

- **Benefits of Screening**: Studies such as the National Lung Screening Trial have shown that LDCT screening can significantly reduce lung cancer mortality in high-risk groups. The main benefit is that it finds cancers at an earlier stage (Stage I or II) when they can be treated more effectively. In fact, early detection via LDCT has been associated with a ~20% reduction in lung cancer death risk in the screened population [8]. Finding cancer before it spreads translates into more lives saved.
- **Risks and Limitations**: Screening is not perfect. Not every cancer will be caught early, and some cancers found early could still be aggressive. Also, LDCT scans often detect nodules or abnormalities that are not cancer (false positives). These can lead to anxiety and additional invasive tests like biopsies or follow-up scans. However, most of these nodules turn out benign. There is also radiation exposure from repeated CT scans (though LDCT uses a lower dose than a standard CT, it's still more than a chest X-ray) [8]. Therefore, screening is a balance of benefit versus risk, and guidelines aim to maximize benefit by targeting those at highest risk (older heavy smokers) [9].

Before starting screening, individuals should have a detailed discussion with their healthcare provider about the potential benefits, risks, and what happens if something abnormal is found [8]. If a screening LDCT shows an abnormal nodule, further evaluation (additional imaging, PET scans, or biopsy) will be needed to determine if it's cancer [8]. It's also crucial that screening is done at experienced centers with multidisciplinary teams, so that abnormalities are properly followed up.

In summary, lung cancer screening with annual low-dose CT is now the standard of care for high-risk populations. This proactive approach is improving early detection: roughly 70% of screen-detected lung cancers are Stage I, which is a huge improvement over the past, where the majority were Stage III or IV at diagnosis. Alongside smoking cessation efforts, screening is a key strategy to reduce lung cancer deaths.

2.4.2 *Staging*

Once lung cancer is diagnosed by biopsy, the next critical step in the diagnostic process is staging determining the extent of disease in the body. Accurate staging informs treatment decisions (for example, whether surgery is feasible, or if chemotherapy/radiation is needed) and provides prognostic information [3]. Lung cancer staging, as described in Sect. 2.1, uses the TNM classification to assign stage 0, I, II, III, or IV. Here we focus on how staging is done in practice.

- **Imaging for Staging**: Several imaging tests are performed:
  - A CT scan of the chest and upper abdomen is standard to evaluate the primary tumor and check for enlarged lymph nodes or adrenal/liver metastases (common spread sites). If not already done, this CT is one of the first staging studies.
  - A PET/CT scan is commonly done for NSCLC staging (and sometimes for limited SCLC). PET/CT can identify metabolically active cancer in lymph nodes or distant organs that might not be obvious on CT. It is very useful for discovering hidden metastases (for instance, a PET might light up a lymph node or a bone lesion, upstaging the cancer) [7].
  - An MRI of the brain is recommended for staging in any patient with sufficiently advanced lung cancer or with symptoms, especially in NSCLC Stage II or higher, and routinely for all SCLC patients, because lung cancer frequently spreads to the brain. As mentioned, MRI is superior to PET for brain imaging [7].
  - Sometimes, other site-specific scans (like an MRI of the spine or a bone scan) may be done if specific symptoms warrant, but PET has largely replaced the need for a dedicated bone scan in NSCLC staging.
- **Invasive Staging (Lymph Node Evaluation)**: Imaging can suggest cancer spread to lymph nodes (for example, a PET-positive mediastinal node), but confirmatory biopsies of lymph nodes are often done for precise staging. Guidelines often

recommend sampling mediastinal lymph nodes before surgery if imaging shows they might be involved [3]. Techniques include:

- **EBUS-TBNA (Endobronchial Ultrasound – Transbronchial Needle Aspiration)**: Performed during bronchoscopy, this uses ultrasound to guide a needle through the airway wall into suspect lymph nodes to get tissue samples [3]. It's minimally invasive and high yield for nodes along the trachea and bronchi.
- **Mediastinoscopy**: A short surgical procedure under general anesthesia where a scope is inserted behind the sternum to biopsy mediastinal lymph nodes directly [3]. This has been a gold standard for decades, allowing direct sampling of nodes in the center of the chest.
- **Thoracoscopy (VATS)** or other surgical methods can sample lymph nodes in certain locations or remove questionable nodes at the time of surgery.
- By obtaining tissue from lymph nodes, doctors can distinguish N0 versus N1 versus N2 disease accurately (no spread to nodes, spread to hilum, or spread to mediastinum, etc.), which determines if surgery is appropriate. For example, confirming cancer in mediastinal nodes (N2) might turn a surgical candidate into a case for chemotherapy and radiation instead. Accurate staging is so important that it is said: "doing the correct treatment depends on getting the staging right" [3].

- **Clinical versus Pathologic Stage**: Initially, patients receive a clinical stage based on all the information gathered before any major treatment (imaging tests, biopsies, etc.) [2]. If the patient then goes to surgery, the removed tumor and lymph nodes are examined by a pathologist, sometimes this reveals more (or less) disease than expected. The final pathologic stage (also called surgical stage) might be adjusted up or down based on what the surgery finds [3]. For instance, clinically a tumor may look like Stage IIA, but if surgery finds tiny metastases in a lymph node that imaging missed, the pathologic stage might be IIIB. Pathologic stage is considered very accurate and is used for final planning (like whether to give post-surgery chemotherapy).

For small cell lung cancer (SCLC), staging with TNM is less emphasized in practice. Often, it's classified simply as limited versus extensive as described in Sect. 2.2. Nonetheless, modern practice does use imaging similarly (CT, PET, MRI) to map SCLC spread. Most SCLC present as extensive stage, so further invasive staging is less frequently needed (because widespread metastases may already be evident, making the point moot). But for a potential limited-stage SCLC, one might do similar lymph node biopsies to ensure it's truly limited.

In summary, staging is about assembling the fullest picture of the cancer's reach. This staging work-up is completed before finalizing the treatment plan. It leverages high-tech imaging and sometimes invasive techniques to sample tissue. The result is an assignment of Stage 0 through IV as previously defined. Treatment strategies in lung cancer hinge on this stage: early-stage (I/II) disease is typically managed with surgery (plus possibly adjuvant therapy), locally advanced (III) often requires combined-modality therapy, and advanced (IV) disease is treated with systemic therapies (see next section). Precision in staging therefore directly impacts patient outcomes [3].

2.5 Treatment for Lung Cancer

Treatment of lung cancer requires a multidisciplinary approach and is tailored to the cancer's type (NSCLC vs. SCLC) and stage, as well as the patient's overall health. Broadly, the main treatment modalities for lung cancer are surgery, chemotherapy, radiation therapy, targeted therapy, and immunotherapy. Often, multiple treatments are used in combination or sequence (multimodal therapy) for the best outcome [9]. For example, a patient with Stage III NSCLC might receive chemotherapy combined with radiation, followed by surgery or immunotherapy, whereas Stage I might be cured with surgery alone. It's also worth noting that treatment approaches differ somewhat between NSCLC and SCLC–NSCLC, especially early-stage, is often surgically managed, whereas SCLC (being usually advanced) is primarily treated with chemoradiation. Below we detail each treatment modality:

2.5.1 Surgery

Surgical resection is the cornerstone treatment for early-stage lung cancers. The goal of surgery is to completely remove the tumor and any affected tissue, offering the best chance for cure localized disease. Surgery is mainly used for NSCLC stages I, II, and some III (and very rarely for a solitary nodule of SCLC, which is uncommon) [4]. If the cancer hasn't spread beyond one lung significantly, a surgeon can operate to excise it. Common surgical procedures include:

- **Lobectomy**: removal of an entire lobe of the lung. (The right lung has 3 lobes, left lung has 2.) This is considered the gold standard for operable NSCLC, as it removes the tumor with a margin and the lung drainage area.
- **Segmentectomy or Wedge Resection**: removal of a part of a lobe. This lung-sparing surgery may be considered for very small cancers or for patients who cannot tolerate a full lobectomy due to limited pulmonary reserve. However, it carries a slightly higher risk of recurrence than lobectomy if used for larger tumors.
- **Pneumonectomy**: removal of an entire lung. This is done if the tumor is centrally located or involves multiple lobes such that a lobectomy would not get it all. Pneumonectomy is a more drastic surgery and only done, if necessary, because of higher morbidity.
- **Lymph Node Dissection or Sampling**: During lung cancer surgery, surgeons also remove nearby lymph nodes from the mediastinum/hilum to check for any spread, which helps accurately stage the disease and guide needs for additional therapy.

Advances in surgical techniques include Video-Assisted Thoracoscopic Surgery (VATS) and robotic-assisted thoracic surgery, which allows lobectomies or wedge resections to be done through small incisions (minimally invasively), reducing recovery time. Regardless of technique, the surgeon aims to remove all visible tumor along with a rim of healthy tissue to ensure clear margins [4].

For early-stage NSCLC, surgery can be curative. Five-year survival rates after resection of stage I NSCLC can exceed 60% [5]. In some cases, surgery may be followed by adjuvant chemotherapy (for stage II or III, to kill any microscopic remaining cancer) or adjuvant immunotherapy (newer protocols for certain high-risk cases). For stage IIIA, sometimes neoadjuvant therapy (chemo or chemoradiation before surgery) is given to shrink the tumor, then surgery. In small cell lung cancer, surgery is rarely an option because SCLC has almost always spread by diagnosis. Only in the rare scenario of a very limited, single small cell tumor (with no spread on PET and negative mediastinal biopsy) would surgery be considered, typically followed by chemo.

The side effects and recovery from lung surgery depend on the extent of resection. Common issues after a lobectomy or pneumonectomy include pain, fatigue, and reduced lung function proportional to how much lung was removed [4]. Many patients experience shortness of breath during recovery but can improve over time as the remaining lung adapts. Pulmonary rehabilitation exercises can help maximize post-surgical lung function. In summary, surgery offers the best chance of long-term survival for localized lung cancer. If the tumor can be completely removed and the patient can tolerate the operation, surgery is usually pursued for stages I-II NSCLC and selected III. The role of surgery diminishes as stage increases, giving way to other modalities for advanced disease.

2.5.2 Chemotherapy

Chemotherapy refers to drugs that kill rapidly dividing cells, and it has long been a mainstay of lung cancer treatment. Chemotherapy is a systemic therapy; the drugs circulate throughout the body to kill cancer cells wherever they may be. In lung cancer, chemotherapy is used in several contexts:

- **Adjuvant Chemotherapy**: After surgery for NSCLC (typically stage II or IIIA), a course of chemo is often given to eradicate microscopic cancer cells and reduce recurrence risk.
- **Neoadjuvant Chemotherapy**: Before surgery (or radiation) to shrink a tumor and improve operability.
- **Concurrent Chemoradiation**: For unresectable Stage III NSCLC or for limited-stage SCLC, chemotherapy is given at the same time as radiation therapy to enhance its effectiveness.

- **First-Line Treatment for Advanced Cancer**: For Stage IV NSCLC (especially if no targetable mutations) and extensive-stage SCLC, chemotherapy is often the primary treatment to control disease and alleviate symptoms.
- **Palliative Chemotherapy**: Even if not curative, chemo can shrink tumors that are causing symptoms (like pain or cough) to improve quality of life.

The chemotherapy regimens for lung cancer usually involve combinations of drugs. In NSCLC, a common backbone is a platinum-based drug (either cisplatin or carboplatin) plus another drug such as paclitaxel, pemetrexed, gemcitabine, or vinorelbine, depending on the subtype and setting. For example, cisplatin + pemetrexed is often used for non-squamous NSCLC, while cisplatin + gemcitabine for squamous NSCLC. In SCLC, the standard has been a platinum (cisplatin or carboplatin) combined with etoposide or irinotecan.

Chemotherapy is typically given in cycles (e.g., every 3 weeks) and often via intravenous infusion. Multiple cycles are required—a usual course might be 4–6 cycles for adjuvant or first-line treatment, but it varies. Chemotherapy works by damaging the DNA or cellular machinery of dividing cells, which is why it can shrink tumors. However, it also affects normal fast-growing cells, leading to side effects. Common side effects of chemotherapy for lung cancer include nausea and vomiting, loss of appetite, hair loss, fatigue, and increased risk of infections due to lowered blood counts [4]. Many of these side effects are manageable with supportive medications (e.g., anti-nausea drugs, growth factors for white blood cells, etc.). Over the past decade, the use of immunotherapy and targeted therapy (see below) has transformed the management of advanced NSCLC, often replacing or supplementing traditional chemo. But even so, chemotherapy remains critical—for instance, immunotherapy is frequently combined with platinum-doublet chemotherapy as an initial treatment in metastatic NSCLC to improve outcomes.

In small cell lung cancer, chemotherapy is essential. SCLC is very chemo-sensitive (responds well initially). The standard regimen for decades has been cisplatin or carboplatin with etoposide. Nearly all SCLC patients, limited or extensive, get chemo; in limited-stage it's combined with radiation, and in extensive-stage it's combined now with immunotherapy (atezolizumab or durvalumab) as the first line, based on recent trials. Without chemo, SCLC prognosis is dismal, as the disease progresses rapidly. With chemo (and radiation in limited stage), remission can often be achieved, though relapses are common.

Overall, chemotherapy has a pivotal role in controlling lung cancer on a systemic level. It has improved survival in all settings of lung cancer when appropriately applied [9]. Newer treatments have augmented the benefits, but chemo is frequently part of combination strategies (e.g., chemo + immunotherapy) for advanced diseases. The decision to use chemotherapy, and which regimen, depends on cancer type, stage, and patient fitness (chemo can be tough on those with frail health). Oncologists weigh these factors to customize the best approach for each patient.

2.5.3 Radiation Therapy

Radiation therapy uses high-energy rays (like X-rays or proton beams) to kill cancer cells or slow their growth. In lung cancer management, radiation is a versatile tool employed in various scenarios:

- **Curative Intent for Early Disease**: For patients with early-stage NSCLC who are not surgical candidates (due to medical comorbidities or refusal of surgery), a specialized form of radiation called stereotactic body radiotherapy (SBRT) can be used to treat small tumors with high doses in a few sessions. SBRT has local control rates approaching those of surgery for small Stage I tumors.
- **Combined with Chemotherapy for Stage III NSCLC**: When surgery isn't possible (e.g., Stage III unresectable cases), concurrent chemoradiation is a standard approach. Radiation is aimed at the lung tumor and involved lymph nodes, while chemotherapy sensitizes the cancer cells to radiation and treats systemic disease. This combination can sometimes cure Stage III disease or at least markedly prolong survival.
- **Post-operative (Adjuvant) Radiation**: In some cases, after surgery, if there are positive margins or residual disease, radiation to the surgical bed or mediastinum may be given to kill remaining cancer cells.
- **Primary Treatment for Limited-Stage SCLC**: In limited-stage small cell lung cancer, radiation to the chest is usually given together with chemotherapy as part of the initial treatment, because SCLC is very radiosensitive [6]. The radiation often starts during cycle 1 or 2 of chemo.
- **Prophylactic Cranial Irradiation (PCI)**: In SCLC, if a patient responds well to initial chemo (and radiation for limited disease), doctors often recommend radiation to the brain (at a low preventive dose). This is because SCLC frequently spreads to the brain, and PCI has been shown to reduce the risk of brain metastases and improve survival in SCLC.
- **Palliation**: Radiation is extremely useful to relieve symptoms caused by lung cancer. For example, radiation can shrink a tumor that's blocking a major airway and causing breathing difficulty [4]. It can be used to alleviate bone pain from metastases or treat brain metastases (with techniques like whole-brain radiation or stereotactic radiosurgery). Palliative radiation focuses on improving quality of life by targeting symptomatic lesions.

Modern radiation therapy techniques for lung cancer include 3D conformal radiation, Intensity-Modulated Radiation Therapy (IMRT), and image-guided approaches that shape beams precisely to the tumor while sparing normal tissues. This is important to minimize damage to lungs (to reduce pneumonitis risk), esophagus (reducing severe esophagitis), heart, and spinal cord. In SBRT for early tumors, very high doses per fraction (session) are delivered with sub-millimeter precision to ablate the tumor in 3–5 treatments.

Common side effects of radiation to the chest can include esophagitis (inflammation of the esophagus causing painful swallowing), radiation pneumonitis (inflammatory reaction in lungs causing cough and shortness of breath, which can occur weeks after treatment), fatigue, skin changes on the chest, and lowered blood counts [4]. These side effects depend on the radiation dose and field. With improved techniques, severe side effects are less common than in the past, but they remain important considerations.

In essence, radiation therapy is a critical component of lung cancer treatment:

- It can eradicate localized tumors (especially with SBRT) when surgery isn't an option.
- It works synergistically with chemotherapy in intermediate stages to attempt cure.
- It provides symptom relief in advanced stages (e.g., relieving pain, bleeding or obstruction).

Because of the risk to vital organs in the chest, radiation planning for lung cancer is quite complex, and specialists carefully balance delivering a tumor-killing dose while protecting as much normal lung as possible [4]. When used appropriately, radiation can significantly improve outcomes in lung cancer, either as part of curative therapy or for palliation.

2.5.4 Targeted Therapy

Targeted therapies are drugs designed to specifically attack cancer cells based on unique molecular features (such as genetic mutations or abnormal proteins) that are driving the cancer's growth. In lung cancer, particularly NSCLC researchers have identified several keys "driver mutations" in subsets of tumors, and drugs have been developed to target those mutated proteins. The result is a form of personalized medicine: if a patient's tumor has a certain mutation, they can receive a drug that precisely targets that molecular abnormality, often yielding dramatic tumor responses. Some of the major targets and corresponding targeted drugs in NSCLC include:

- **EGFR Mutations**: About 10–15% of NSCLC (especially adenocarcinoma in non-smokers, Asians) have mutations in the EGFR gene. EGFR inhibitors (like erlotinib, gefitinib, afatinib, and the newer Osimertinib) block the epidermal growth factor receptor pathway that the mutant cells depend on [10]. These pills often cause tumors to shrink significantly in patients with EGFR-mutant lung cancer and are a standard first-line treatment for such cases, with better tolerability than chemo.
- **PIK3CA Mutations**: studies have shown hot spot mutations of pik3ca genes are responsible for number of cancers and nowadays kinase inhibitors are used to treat the cancer [11–13].

- **ALK Rearrangements**: A smaller fraction (around 5%) of NSCLC has a fusion of the ALK gene. ALK inhibitors (crizotinib was first, newer ones like alcedinid, lorlatinib, etc. are more potent) can produce high response rates in ALK-positive lung cancer and improve survival. Similarly, ROS1 gene fusions (around 1–2%) are treated with some of the ALK/ROS1 inhibitors [10].
- **KRAS Mutations**: KRAS is one of the most common mutations in lung adenocarcinoma (~25–30%), especially in smokers. For a long time it was "undruggable," but recently new drugs targeting a specific subtype (KRAS G12C mutation) like sotorasib have become available.
- **BRAF V600E Mutations**: (1–2% of lung adenocarcinoma) can be treated with BRAF inhibitors (dabrafenib) plus MEK inhibitors (trametinib), borrowing from melanoma treatments.
- MET exon 14 skipping mutations, RET fusions, NTRK fusions, HER2 mutations, etc. are other less common drivers, each now has matched targeted therapies (e.g., MET inhibitors like capmatinib, RET inhibitors like selpercatinib, TRK inhibitors, etc.).

The effect of targeted therapy can be profound; patients often see rapid symptom improvement and tumor shrinkage if their tumor harbors the target. These drugs tend to be oral medications taken daily. They also often have different side effect profiles than traditional chemo for example, EGFR inhibitors commonly cause skin rash and diarrhea, ALK inhibitors can cause liver enzyme changes, vision changes, or swelling, etc., but generally they don't cause the hair loss or severe nausea that chemo does [10]. However, tumors can develop resistance to targeted drugs over time (through new mutations or alternate pathways), so responses may last on the order of months to a few years before the cancer finds a way to grow again.

Targeted therapies are mainly used in advanced/metastatic NSCLC (Stage IV) as first-line treatment if a driver mutation is present, because they can prolong life and are often better tolerated than chemo. Increasingly, some targeted drugs are also being tested in earlier stages (e.g., adjuvant osimertinib for EGFR-mutant stage IB-III after surgery showed improved disease-free survival). For instance, osimertinib is now approved as an adjuvant therapy after surgery and chemo for EGFR-mutant NSCLC, to reduce recurrence [10].

In small cell lung cancer, targeted therapy has had less success because SCLC typically doesn't have the same actionable mutations as NSCLC (it's often driven by loss of tumor suppressor genes like TP53 and RB1, which we cannot directly target yet). Research is ongoing for SCLC targeted approaches.

Overall, the advent of targeted therapy has marked a revolution in lung cancer treatment. It exemplifies the importance of doing molecular testing on biopsy samples (as mentioned in Sect. 2.3.1). By matching the right drug to the right patient, outcomes have improved. For example, patients with EGFR-mutant NSCLC have significantly longer median survival on EGFR inhibitors compared to old chemotherapy regimens [10]. As science discovers more about tumor genomics, the list of targets and corresponding drugs continues to grow (e.g., newer targets like HER2 mutations, KRAS G12C as mentioned, etc. now have therapies in clinical use [10]).

2.5.5 Immunotherapy

Immunotherapy is another breakthrough approach that has transformed lung cancer treatment in the past decade. Unlike chemotherapy which directly kills cancer cells, immunotherapy works by empowering the patient's own immune system to recognize and destroy cancer cells [4]. The most successful immunotherapies for lung cancer have been the immune checkpoint inhibitors, which target inhibitory pathways that cancers use to hide from immune attack. The key drugs are:

- PD-1 inhibitors (Programmed Death-1 inhibitors) such as nivolumab and pembrolizumab.
- PD-L1 inhibitors (targeting the ligand PD-L1 on tumor cells) such as atezolizumab and durvalumab.
- (Less commonly in lung cancer) CTLA-4 inhibitors like ipilimumab, sometimes used in combination with PD-1 blockers.

These checkpoint inhibitors basically unblock the immune system. Many tumors express PD-L1 which bind PD-1 on T-cells and turn them off. Drugs like pembrolizumab block this interaction, so the T-cells stay active and can attack the cancer. In lung cancer, trials showed that in patients with high PD-L1 expression on their tumors, pembrolizumab alone was better than chemotherapy as first-line treatment, and even in unselected patients, adding pembrolizumab to chemo improved survival [4]. Consequently, immunotherapy is now part of standard first-line therapy for most advanced NSCLC (either alone or with chemo, depending on PD-L1 level). For example:

- **Advanced NSCLC**: Pembrolizumab is often given in combination with platinum-doublet chemotherapy for first-line treatment (for non-squamous, along with pemetrexed; for squamous, with taxane, etc.) [4]. If the tumor has very high PD-L1 ($\geq$50%), pembrolizumab might even be used alone initially. Nivolumab and atezolizumab are also used in various lines of therapy.
- **Stage III NSCLC (Unresectable)**: After concurrent chemoradiation, giving 1 year of durvalumab (a PD-L1 inhibitor) as consolidation therapy significantly improved survival (the PACIFIC trial), this is now a standard of care for Stage III that did not progress after chemoradiation.
- **Extensive-Stage SCLC**: Adding atezolizumab or durvalumab to first-line chemo (platinum + etoposide) was shown to improve survival in extensive SCLC, so now immunotherapy is included in frontline SCLC as well.

Immunotherapy can produce long-lasting remissions in a subset of patients, something rarely seen with chemo alone. There are patients with metastatic lung cancer alive many years later after immunotherapy, essentially a rarity prior to these drugs. However, only a portion of patients respond, and we don't fully understand why some do and some don't (beyond PD-L1 levels and other biomarkers).

Side effects of immunotherapy are distinct from chemo. Because these drugs stimulate the immune system, they can cause inflammatory side effects known as immune-related adverse events. Common ones include rash and itching, thyroid gland dysfunction, hepatitis, colitis (causing diarrhea), pneumonitis (inflammation of lungs), and others [4]. These can often be managed with corticosteroids or immunosuppressants if recognized early, and most patients don't experience severe issues. Generally, immunotherapy is better tolerated than cytotoxic chemo for many patients. Immunotherapy is an active area of research in lung cancer, including combining multiple immunotherapies or using them in earlier stages (e.g., neoadjuvant immunotherapy before surgery is being studied, and one combination of nivolumab + chemo pre-surgery has already been approved for resectable NSCLC based on improved pathologic response rates).

In summary, checkpoint immunotherapy has become a pillar of lung cancer treatment, especially for NSCLC. It works by taking the "brakes" off the immune system, allowing T-cells to attack the cancer [4]. This has yielded significant improvements in survival for many patients with advanced disease and is now part of standard care in both metastatic NSCLC and SCLC (extensive stage), as well as a consolidation after Stage III chemoradiation. Ongoing studies are expanding its role, and newer forms of immunotherapy (like CAR-T cells or cancer vaccines) are being explored for the future. CRISPR/cas9 therapy might be useful to treat cancer at early stage [14].

2.6 Summary

The landscape of lung cancer therapy has evolved considerably. Early-stage lung cancer can often be cured with surgery (or stereotactic radiation), whereas locally advanced disease requires a combination of chemotherapy, radiation, and sometimes surgery. Metastatic lung cancer, once nearly uniformly fatal within a year, can now often be managed chronically for several years thanks to targeted pills and immunotherapy that were not available a decade ago. Nonetheless, lung cancer remains a formidable disease prevention (smoking cessation) and early detection (screening) are crucial public health strategies to reduce its impact. By understanding the types of lung cancer, how to diagnose and stage it accurately, and how to deploy the array of modern treatments, clinicians aim to improve survival and quality of life for patients facing this challenging cancer.

References

1. Lung cancer facts. Website: https://www.lungcancerresearchfoundation.org/for-patients/lung-cancer-facts/. Last Access: February 2026.
2. Non-small Cell Lung Cancer Stages. Website: https://www.cancer.org/cancer/types/lung-cancer/detection-diagnosis-staging/staging-nsclc.html. Last Access: February 2026.
3. Lung Cancer Staging. Website: https://www.lung.org/lung-health-diseases/lung-disease-lookup/lung-cancer/symptoms-diagnosis/lung-cancer-staging. Last Access: February 2026.

4. Lung Cancer. Website: https://my.clevelandclinic.org/health/diseases/4375-lung-cancer. Last Access: February 2026.
5. Lung Cancer Survival Rates. Website: https://www.cancer.org/cancer/types/lung-cancer/detection-diagnosis-staging/survival-rates.html. Last Access: February 2026.
6. What is Lung Cancer? Website: https://www.cancer.org/cancer/types/lung-cancer/about/what-is.html. Last Access: February 2026.
7. Tests for Lung Cancer. Website: https://www.cancer.org/cancer/types/lung-cancer/detection-diagnosis-staging/how-diagnosed.html. Last Access: February 2026.
8. Can Lung cancer be found early? Website: https://www.cancer.org/cancer/types/lung-cancer/detection-diagnosis-staging/detection.html. Last Access: February 2026.
9. Lung Cancer: Screening. Website: https://www.uspreventiveservicestaskforce.org/uspstf/recommendation/lung-cancer-screening. Last Access: February 2026.
10. Targeted Drug Therapy for Non-small Cell Lung Cancer. Website: https://www.cancer.org/cancer/types/lung-cancer/treating-non-small-cell/targeted-therapies.html. Last Access: February 2026.
11. Shah, S., Shah, S., Padh, H., & Kalia, K. (2015). Genetic alterations of the PIK3CA oncogene in human oral squamous cell carcinoma in an Indian population. *Oral Surgery, Oral Medicine, Oral Pathology and Oral Radiology, 120*(5), 628–635.
12. Patel, A., Mahapatra, S., Bishoyi, A. K., Sharma, A., Makwana, A., Swarnkar, T., Gupta, A., Sahoo, P. K., & Shah, S. (2025). Harnessing machine learning technique to authenticate differentially expressed genes in oral squamous cell carcinoma. *Oral Surgery, Oral Medicine, Oral Pathology and Oral Radiology, 139*(2), 211–219.
13. Shah, S., Mishra, G., & Kalia, K. (2018). Single nucleotide polymorphism rs17849071 G/T in the PIK3CA gene is inversely associated with oral cancer. *Oral Cancer, 2*(3), 83–89.
14. Nalla, Y., & Shah, S. (2021). A new era in molecular biology clustered regularly interspaced short palindromic repeats/cas9 technology: A brief understanding. *Advances in Human Biology, 11*(2), 152–156.

Chapter 3
Artificial Intelligence and Its Role in Early Detection of Lung Cancer

Lung cancer is responsible for more cancer-related deaths globally than any other malignancy, accounting for approximately 1.8 million deaths annually [1]. Survival outcomes are strongly associated with disease stage at diagnosis, with five-year survival rates exceeding 60% for stage I disease compared to fewer than 10% for metastatic presentations [2]. This stark disparity underscores the clinical imperative for effective early detection. Artificial intelligence (AI), particularly deep learning-based medical imaging analysis, has emerged as a transformative paradigm promising to extend the reach and accuracy of lung cancer screening beyond what is achievable with conventional radiological review alone.

3.1 Artificial Intelligence (AI)

Artificial intelligence is a broad field of computer science concerned with the design of systems that can perform tasks normally requiring human cognition [3]. The contemporary resurgence of AI is largely attributable to three converging factors: the availability of large-scale digital datasets, the proliferation of high-performance parallel computing hardware, and methodological advances in deep neural network architectures [4].

AI encompasses a hierarchy of subfields. Machine learning (ML) refers to the capacity of algorithms to improve through experience without being explicitly programmed [5]. Deep learning (DL) employs artificial neural networks with multiple layers to model complex, high-dimensional data such as medical images [6]. Natural language processing (NLP) enables machines to understand and generate human language, facilitating analysis of clinical notes and radiology reports [7]. Computer vision provides the algorithmic foundations for interpreting visual data, including CT volumes and histopathology whole-slide images [8]. Table 3.1 shows core AI components and their applications in medicine field.

S. Shah and R. Thanki, *Artificial Intelligence for Early Detection and Diagnosis of Lung Cancer*, Signals and Communication Technology,
https://doi.org/10.1007/978-3-032-29615-3_3

Table 3.1 Core AI components and their applications in medicine

AI component	Definition	Medical application examples
Machine learning (ML)	Statistical algorithms that learn from data without explicit programming	SVM, Random Forests, XGBoost; EHR-based risk scoring [5]
Deep learning (DL)	Multi-layer neural networks extracting hierarchical features automatically	CNNs, RNNs, Transformers; dominant in medical imaging [6]
Natural language processing (NLP)	Computational methods for understanding and generating human language	Clinical note parsing, radiology report mining [7]
Computer vision (CV)	Algorithms enabling machines to interpret visual data	Nodule detection, tumor segmentation, histopathology [8]
Reinforcement learning (RL)	Agents learn by maximizing cumulative reward through trial and error	Treatment planning optimization, adaptive CDSS
Generative AI	Models that synthesize realistic data to augment scarce medical datasets	GANs, VAEs, diffusion models for synthetic CT/PET generation

3.2 AI in Healthcare Research

The integration of AI into healthcare research has accelerated markedly, with annual publications growing from fewer than 500 in 2010 to more than 20,000 by 2022 [9, 10]. AI has demonstrated competencies across biomedical imaging, drug discovery, genomic analysis, clinical decision support, and hospital operations [11, 12]. CNNs have achieved performance comparable to or exceeding expert clinicians in tasks such as skin lesion classification [13], diabetic retinopathy grading [14], and chest radiograph interpretation [15]. As of 2023, the FDA had authorized 692 AI/ML-enabled medical devices, of which approximately 75% were radiology-related [16] (Table 3.2).

3.3 Role of AI in Cancer Detection

Cancer detection presents an ideal use-case for AI because the task is predominantly perceptual and pattern-recognition-based, large, labeled imaging datasets exist [17], and the consequences of missed diagnoses are severe [18]. AI systems serve principally as computer-aided detection (CADe) or computer-aided diagnosis (CADx) systems, or as multimodal data integrators delivering end-to-end risk stratification [19, 20]. Key performance metrics include sensitivity, specificity, positive predictive value (PPV), negative predictive value (NPV), and the area under the receiver

Table 3.2 AI applications across healthcare research domains

Domain	Key task	AI methods
Medical imaging	Radiograph, CT, MRI, PET analysis	CNNs, U-Net, Vision Transformers
Drug discovery	Target identification, virtual screening	Graph Neural Networks, DL-QSAR
Clinical decision support	Diagnosis, triage, treatment aid	Ensemble classifiers, rule-based ML
Genomics and precision medicine	Variant calling, cancer subtyping	Deep learning on omics data
Electronic health records	Outcome prediction, risk scoring	LSTM, BERT-based NLP
Pathology	Tissue classification, grading	Whole-slide image CNNs
Robotic surgery	Autonomous task assistance	Reinforcement learning, CV

operating characteristic curve (AUC-ROC) [21]. A clinically deployable AI system must achieve not only high sensitivity but also acceptably low false-positive rates to prevent unnecessary downstream investigations (Fig. 3.1).

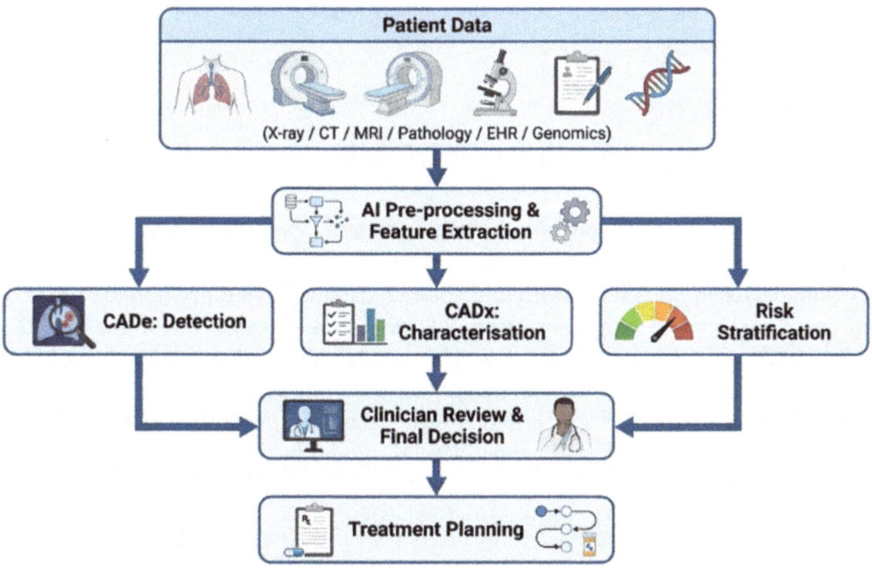

Fig. 3.1 Generalized AI-enabled workflow for cancer detection

3.4 Roles of AI in Detection and Diagnosis of Lung Cancer

Lung cancer detection encompasses a cascade of clinical tasks, from population-level risk assessment through radiological screening, nodule characterization, histological classification, and staging. AI contributes meaningfully at each stage [11, 18]. The following subsections delineate the principal functional roles.

3.4.1 Automated Image Analysis

The most widely studied AI application is the automated analysis of low-dose CT (LDCT) images, the only screening modality shown to reduce lung cancer mortality in high-risk populations [22, 23]. CNNs trained on large, annotated CT datasets, most notably the NLST and LIDC-IDRI have demonstrated the capacity to detect pulmonary nodules with sensitivities exceeding 95% [24, 25]. Three-dimensional convolutional architectures process volumetric CT data, capturing spatial relationships across axial, coronal, and sagittal planes. Multi-scale and attention-based models improve detection of small (< 6 mm) and ground-glass opacity (GGO) nodules [26]. Importantly, AI systems operate consistently without fatigue or cognitive biases affecting human performance under high-volume reporting conditions [27].

3.4.2 Computer-Aided Diagnosis (CAD)

CAD systems integrate detection with characterization, providing malignancy probability estimates by combining CNN-derived imaging features with radiomic descriptors quantitative metrics such as nodule volume, density, sphericity, and texture [28]. Radiomics-augmented deep learning models have demonstrated AUC values of 0.92–0.99 in retrospective studies, outperforming radiologist stratification based on Lung-RADS criteria alone [27, 29]. Temporal analysis comparing current and prior CT scans to assess nodule growth kinetics represents an additional AI-based CADx capability. Ardila et al. demonstrated that a DL model incorporating prior CT information achieved an AUC of 0.944 on the NLST dataset, reducing false-positive rates by 11% compared to expert radiologists [24] (Table 3.3).

3.4.3 Risk Stratification

Beyond individual lesion characterization, AI enables population-level risk stratification by integrating imaging features with clinical risk factors such as age, smoking

Table 3.3 Landmark computer-aided diagnosis (CAD) systems for lung cancer

CAD system	Primary task	Architecture	Performance/Citation
NoduleX	CT-based pulmonary nodule detection	Ensemble of CNNs and random forest	Sensitivity 97.4%, AUC 0.99 [25]
Lung-RADS AI	Nodule risk categorization (ACR Lung-RADS)	U-Net + risk classifier	Radiologist concordance ~ 91% [30]
Sybil	6-year lung cancer risk from single LDCT	3D CNN on LDCT slices	AUC 0.86–0.94 [31]
Google DeepMind	Malignancy prediction from LDCT	3D DL with prior CT integration	Accuracy 94.4%; 11% fewer FP [24]
InferRead CT Lung	Commercial CADe/ CADx system	Multi-scale deep CNN	CE-marked; sensitivity 95% + [27]

history, family history, occupational exposures, and COPD status [32]. The Sybil model predicts six-year lung cancer risk from a single LDCT scan with an AUC of 0.75–0.86, enabling precision-targeted screening recall intervals rather than annual uniform recall [28].

3.4.4 Integration with Electronic Health Records (EHR)

EHR data comprising structured fields and unstructured clinical narratives constitute a rich resource for AI-driven lung cancer detection. NLP algorithms applied to free-text radiology reports can extract incidental nodule findings not formally communicated to ordering clinicians, closing a well-documented gap in the follow-up care pathway [33]. FHIR-compliant APIs enable real-time bidirectional data exchange between AI inference engines and hospital EHR systems [34].

3.4.5 Prediction Models

AI-based prediction models span three principal categories: (1) incidence prediction models estimating future lung cancer probability; (2) diagnostic classification models distinguishing malignant from benign lesions; and (3) prognostic models predicting recurrence-free survival, overall survival, or treatment response [20, 35]. Survival prediction models based on DeepSurv have achieved concordance indices (C-index) of 0.70–0.78 in NSCLC cohorts [36].

3.4.6 Mobile Health (mHealth) Solutions

The deployment of AI within mobile health platforms has opened the prospect of extending lung cancer screening to low- and middle-income countries (LMICs) where access to CT scanners and specialist radiologists is constrained. Federated learning, a distributed AI training paradigm enabling model development without sharing raw patient data enables robust mHealth models without compromising patient privacy [30, 37].

3.5 Various Stages of Detection and Diagnosis of Lung Cancer Using AI

The clinical pathway from initial suspicion to definitive lung cancer diagnosis and management involves multiple discrete stages, each presenting opportunities for AI-assisted decision support [18]. Figure 3.2 shows various stages of AI-assisted lung cancer detection and diagnosis. Table 3.4 shows AI roles across the lung cancer detection and management continuum.

3.5.1 Screening and Triage

Population-level screening with LDCT is recommended for high-risk individuals (age 50–80, $\geq$ 20 pack-year smoking history; USPSTF 2021). AI triage systems applied to screening programs identify CTs that can be cleared as normal without immediate radiologist review, and flag high-suspicion cases for expedited assessment. Studies have demonstrated that AI triaging can safely defer approximately 30–50% of routine LDCT reads [24]. The Lung-RADS classification system has been augmented by AI models that automate category assignment, reducing inter-reader variability [44].

3.5.2 Histopathology Image Analysis

Pathological classification underpins treatment selection. AI applied to digitized H&E-stained whole-slide images (WSIs) has demonstrated the capacity to distinguish NSCLC subtypes lung adenocarcinoma (LUAD) versus squamous cell carcinoma (LUSC) with accuracies of 92–97% [39]. DL models trained on WSIs can additionally predict molecular alterations EGFR mutation, ALK rearrangement, PD-L1 expression directly from H&E images [40]. Vision Transformer and multi-instance learning (MIL) frameworks have proven particularly effective for WSI analysis [38].

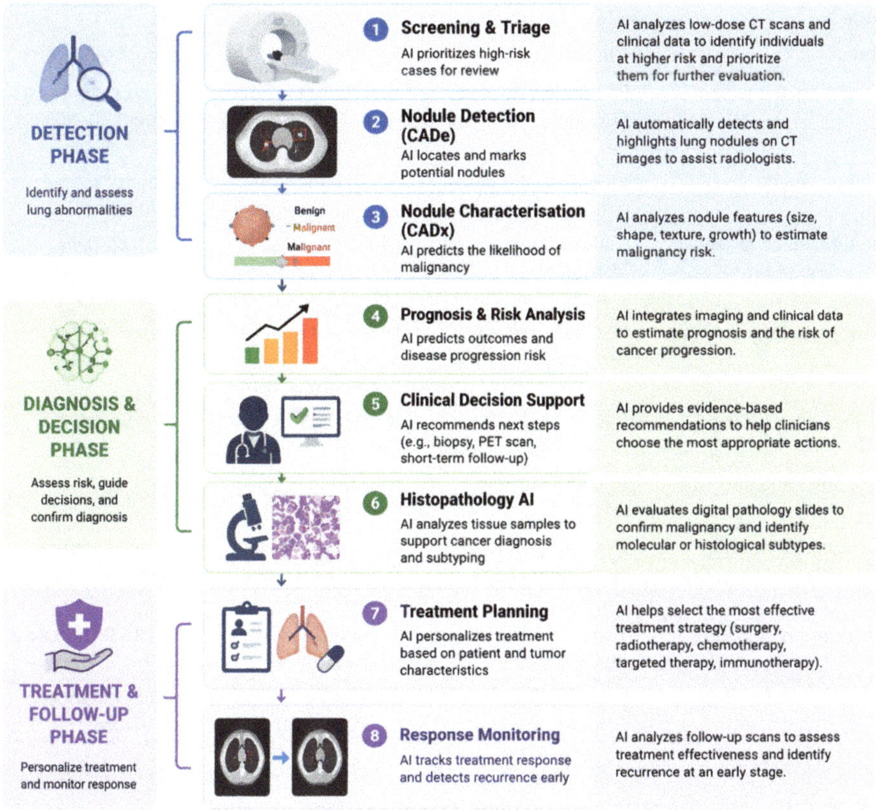

Fig. 3.2 Sequential stages of AI-assisted lung cancer detection and diagnosis

3.5.3 Prognosis and Risk Analysis

Following diagnosis, AI models contribute to prognostic stratification by integrating imaging, pathological, molecular, and clinical data. Radiogenomics approaches identify CT imaging correlates of underlying genomic alterations, enabling non-invasive tumor characterization [35]. Multimodal prognostic frameworks combining DL-extracted CT radiomic features with pathology image features and clinical covariates have achieved C-index values of 0.74–0.78 in external validation cohorts [20, 35].

Table 3.4 AI roles across the lung cancer detection and management continuum

Stage	Clinical goal	Key AI tools	Reported outcomes
Screening and triage	Population-level risk filtering	LDCT + AI risk score (Sybil [31], InferRead [27])	Reduces radiologist workload 30–50%
Nodule detection	Identify and localized pulmonary nodules	3D CNN (NoduleX [25], DeepMed)	Sensitivity > 95%; specificity > 85%
Nodule characterization	Classify malignancy likelihood	Multi-task DL, radiomics fusion [31]	AUC 0.92–0.99
Histopathology analysis	NSCLC vs SCLC subtyping, grading	WSI-CNN (ResNet, Vision Transformer) [38]	Accuracy 92–97% [39]
Molecular profiling	Predict EGFR/ALK/PD-L1 from imaging	Radiogenomics DL [40]	Emerging; AUC ~ 0.80
Prognosis and survival	Predict recurrence and OS	Multimodal DL + Cox-PH [36]	C-index 0.70–0.78 [35]
Treatment planning	Dose optimization, target delineation	RL + GAN-augmented planning [41]	Reduces planning time by 60%
Response monitoring	Tumor volume change over therapy	Longitudinal 3D segmentation [42]	mRECIST alignment > 90%
Clinical decision support	Integrate evidence at point of care	Knowledge graph + NLP + ML [43]	Reduces diagnostic error ~ 15%

3.5.4 Treatment Planning and Response Monitoring

AI contributes to radiation therapy planning through automated tumor and organ-at-risk (OAR) delineation. AI-based segmentation employing 3D U-Net or Swin-UNETR architectures can reduce contouring time by up to 60% while achieving Dice similarity coefficients of 0.82–0.89 [41]. AI-driven longitudinal tumor segmentation enables automated, objective measurement of tumor burden dynamics according to RECIST 1.1 criteria [42].

3.5.5 Clinical Decision Support

Clinical decision support systems (CDSS) powered by AI aggregate evidence from imaging, pathology, genomics, clinical guidelines, and the patient's individual record. Natural language generation models can produce draft structured radiology reports, reducing reporting time by approximately 30% [45]. Knowledge graph-based CDSS integrating medical ontologies with ML-derived clinical insights can provide contextualized differential diagnoses, potentially reducing diagnostic error rates by up to 15% [43].

3.6 Summary

This chapter explains the transformative role of artificial intelligence (AI) in the early detection and diagnosis of lung cancer, the leading cause of cancer-related deaths globally. It highlights the importance of early detection, as survival rates are significantly higher for stage I disease compared to advanced stages. AI, particularly deep learning, has revolutionized medical imaging analysis, enabling more accurate and efficient lung cancer screening. The chapter delves into various AI subfields, including machine learning, deep learning, natural language processing, computer vision, reinforcement learning, and generative AI, and their applications in healthcare. It emphasizes AI's contributions to cancer detection, such as computer-aided detection (CADe), computer-aided diagnosis (CADx), risk stratification, integration with electronic health records (EHR), and prediction models. AI systems have demonstrated high sensitivity and specificity in detecting pulmonary nodules, characterizing malignancy, and predicting cancer risk and survival outcomes. The chapter also discusses AI's role in histopathology analysis, treatment planning, response monitoring, and clinical decision support, showcasing its potential to reduce diagnostic errors, improve efficiency, and enhance patient outcomes. AI's integration into mobile health platforms is highlighted as a promising solution for extending lung cancer screening to underserved regions. Overall, the chapter underscores AI's pivotal role in advancing lung cancer detection, diagnosis, and management across various stages of care.

References

1. World Health Organization. Global cancer observatory: Cancer today. Lyon: IARC; 2023. Available from: https://gco.iarc.fr/today. Last Access: March 2026.
2. Siegel, R. L., Miller, K. D., Wagle, N. S., & Jemal, A. (2023). Cancer statistics, 2023. *CA: A Cancer Journal for Clinicians, 73*(1), 17–48.
3. Russell, S., & Norvig, P. (2002). Artificial intelligence: A modern approach. 592.
4. LeCun, Y., Bengio, Y., & Hinton, G. (2015). Deep learning. *Nature, 521*(7553), 436–444.
5. Ayodele, T. O. (2010). Machine learning overview. *New Advances in Machine Learning, 2*(9–18), 16.
6. Goodfellow, I., Bengio, Y., Courville, A., & Bengio, Y. (2016). *Deep learning* (Vol. 1, No. 2, pp. 1–800). MIT Press.
7. Jiang, F., Jiang, Y., Zhi, H., Dong, Y., Li, H., Ma, S., Wang, Y., Dong, Q., Shen, H., & Wang, Y. (2017). Artificial intelligence in healthcare: Past, present and future. *Stroke and Vascular Neurology*, *2*(4).
8. Shen, D., Wu, G., & Suk, H. I. (2017). Deep learning in medical image analysis. *Annual Review of Biomedical Engineering, 19*, 221–248.

9. Davenport, T., & Kalakota, R. (2019). The potential for artificial intelligence in healthcare. *Future Healthcare Journal, 6*(2), 94–98.
10. Briganti, G., & Le Moine, O. (2020). Artificial intelligence in medicine: Today and tomorrow. *Frontiers in Medicine, 7*, Article 509744.
11. Topol, E. J. (2019). High-performance medicine: The convergence of human and artificial intelligence. *Nature Medicine, 25*(1), 44–56.
12. Rajkomar, A., Oren, E., Chen, K., Dai, A. M., Hajaj, N., Hardt, M., Liu, P.J., Liu, X., Marcus, J., Sun, M., et al. (2018). Scalable and accurate deep learning with electronic health records. *NPJ Digital Medicine, 1*(1), 18.
13. Esteva, A., Kuprel, B., Novoa, R. A., Ko, J., Swetter, S. M., Blau, H. M., & Thrun, S. (2017). Dermatologist-level classification of skin cancer with deep neural networks. *Nature, 542*(7639), 115–118.
14. Gulshan, V., Peng, L., Coram, M., Stumpe, M. C., Wu, D., Narayanaswamy, A., Venugopalan, S., Widner, K., Madams, T., Cuadros, J., Kim, R., Raman, R., Nelson, P. C., Mega, J. L., & Webster, D. R. (2016). Development and validation of a deep learning algorithm for detection of diabetic retinopathy in retinal fundus photographs. *JAMA, 316*(22), 2402–2410.
15. Rajpurkar, P., Irvin, J., Zhu, K., Yang, B., Mehta, H., Duan, T., Bagul, A., Langlotz, C., Shpanskaya, K., Lungren, M. P., & Ng, A. Y. (2017). Chexnet: Radiologist-level pneumonia detection on chest x-rays with deep learning. arXiv preprint arXiv:1711.05225
16. Hill, D. L. (2024). AI in imaging: The regulatory landscape. *British Journal of Radiology, 97*(1155), 483–491.
17. Clark, K., Vendt, B., Smith, K., Freymann, J., Kirby, J., Koppel, P., Moore, S., Phillips, S., Maffitt, D., Pringle, M., et al. (2013). The Cancer Imaging Archive (TCIA): maintaining and operating a public information repository. *Journal of Digital Imaging, 26*(6), 1045–1057.
18. Bi, W. L., Hosny, A., Schabath, M. B., Giger, M. L., Birkbak, N. J., Mehrtash, A., et al. (2019). Artificial intelligence in cancer imaging: clinical challenges and applications. *CA: A Cancer Journal for Clinicians, 69*(2), 127–157.
19. Kather, J. N., Krisam, J., Charoentong, P., Luedde, T., Herpel, E., Weis, C. A., Gaiser, T., Marx, A., Valous, N. A., Ferber, D., et al. (2019). Predicting survival from colorectal cancer histology slides using deep learning: A retrospective multicenter study. *PLoS Medicine, 16*(1), e1002730.
20. Xu, Y., Hosny, A., Zeleznik, R., Parmar, C., Coroller, T., Franco, I., Mak, R. J., & Aerts, H. J. (2019). Deep learning predicts lung cancer treatment response from serial medical imaging. *Clinical Cancer Research, 25*(11), 3266–3275.
21. Parikh, R. B., Teeple, S., & Navathe, A. S. (2019). Addressing bias in artificial intelligence in health care. *JAMA, 322*(24), 2377–2378.
22. National Lung Screening Trial Research Team. (2011). Reduced lung-cancer mortality with low-dose computed tomographic screening. *New England Journal of Medicine, 365*(5), 395–409.
23. de Koning, H. J., van Der Aalst, C. M., de Jong, P. A., Scholten, E. T., Nackaerts, K., Heuvelmans, M. A., Lammers, J. W. J., Weenink, C., Yousaf-Khan, U., Horeweg, N., Westeinde, S. V., Prokop, M., Mali, W. P., Mohamed Hoesein, F. A. A., van Ooijen, P. M. A., Aerts, J. G. J. V., den Bakker, M. A., Thunnissen, E., Verschakelen, J., … Oudkerk, M. (2020). Reduced lung-cancer mortality with volume CT screening in a randomized trial. *New England Journal of Medicine, 382*(6), 503–513.
24. Ardila, D., Kiraly, A. P., Bharadwaj, S., Choi, B., Reicher, J. J., Peng, L., Tse, D., Etemadi, M., Ye, W., Corrado, G., Naidich, D. P., & Shetty, S. (2019). End-to-end lung cancer screening with three-dimensional deep learning on low-dose chest computed tomography. *Nature Medicine, 25*(6), 954–961.
25. Causey, J. L., Zhang, J., Ma, S., Jiang, B., Qualls, J. A., Politte, D. G., Prior, F., Zhang, S., & Huang, X. (2018). Highly accurate model for prediction of lung nodule malignancy with CT scans. *Scientific Reports, 8*(1), 9286.
26. Jin, H., Yu, C., Zhang, J., Zheng, R., Fu, Y., & Zhao, Y. (2025). Multitask Swin Transformer for classification and characterization of pulmonary nodules in CT images. *Quantitative Imaging in Medicine and Surgery, 15*(3), 1845–1861.

27. Guo, Y., Song, Q., Jiang, M., Guo, Y., Xu, P., Zhang, Y., Fang, Q., Zeng, M., & Yao, X. (2021). Histological subtypes classification of lung cancers on CT images using 3D deep learning and radiomics. *Academic Radiology*, *28*(9), e258–e266.
28. Lambin, P., Leijenaar, R. T., Deist, T. M., Peerlings, J., De Jong, E. E., Van Timmeren, J., Sanduleanu, S., Larue, R. T., Even, A. J., Jochems, A., et al. (2017). Radiomics: The bridge between medical imaging and personalized medicine. *Nature Reviews Clinical Oncology*, *14*(12), 749–762.
29. McWilliams, A., Tammemagi, M. C., Mayo, J. R., Roberts, H., Liu, G., Soghrati, K., Yasufuku, K., Martel, S., Laberge, F., Gingras, M., et al. (2013). Probability of cancer in pulmonary nodules detected on first screening CT. *New England Journal of Medicine*, *369*(10), 910–919.
30. McMahan, B., Moore, E., Ramage, D., Hampson, S., & y Arcas, B. A. (2017, April). Communication-efficient learning of deep networks from decentralized data. In *Artificial intelligence and statistics* (pp. 1273–1282). Pmlr.
31. Mikhael, P. G., Wohlwend, J., Yala, A., Karstens, L., Xiang, J., Takigami, A. K., Bourgouin, P. P., Chan, P., Mrah, S., Amayri, W., Juan, Y.-H., Yang, C.-T., Wan, Y.-L., Lin, G., Sequist, L. V., Fintelmann, F. J., & Barzilay, R. (2023). Sybil: A validated deep learning model to predict future lung cancer risk from a single low-dose chest computed tomography. *Journal of Clinical Oncology*, *41*(12), 2191–2200.
32. Tammemägi, M. C., Katki, H. A., Hocking, W. G., Church, T. R., Caporaso, N., Kvale, P. A., Chaturvedi, A. K., Silvestri, G. A., Riley, T. L., Commins, J., & Berg, C. D. (2013). Selection criteria for lung-cancer screening. *New England Journal of Medicine*, *368*(8), 728–736.
33. Pham, A. D., Névéol, A., Lavergne, T., Yasunaga, D., Clément, O., Meyer, G., Morello, R., & Burgun, A. (2014). Natural language processing of radiology reports for the detection of thromboembolic diseases and clinically relevant incidental findings. *BMC Bioinformatics*, *15*(1), 266.
34. HL7 International. HL7 FHIR Release 4.0. 2021. Available from: https://www.hl7.org/fhir/R4/. Last Access: March 2026.
35. Bakr, S., Gevaert, O., Echegaray, S., Ayers, K., Zhou, M., Shafiq, M., Zheng, H., Benson, J. A., Zhang, W., Leung, A. N., et al. (2018). A radiogenomic dataset of non-small cell lung cancer. *Scientific Data*, *5*(1), 180202.
36. Katzman, J. L., Shaham, U., Cloninger, A., Bates, J., Jiang, T., & Kluger, Y. (2018). DeepSurv: Personalized treatment recommender system using a Cox proportional hazards deep neural network. *BMC Medical Research Methodology*, *18*(1), 24.
37. Rieke, N., Hancox, J., Li, W., Milletari, F., Roth, H. R., Albarqouni, S., Bakas, S., Galtier, M. N., Landman, B. A., Maier-Hein, K., Ourselin, S., et al. (2020). The future of digital health with federated learning. *NPJ Digital Medicine*, *3*(1), 119.
38. Chen, R. J., Chen, C., Li, Y., Chen, T. Y., Trister, A. D., Krishnan, R. G., & Mahmood, F. (2022). Scaling vision transformers to gigapixel images via hierarchical self-supervised learning. In *Proceedings of the IEEE/CVF conference on computer vision and pattern recognition* (pp. 16144–16155).
39. Coudray, N., Ocampo, P. S., Sakellaropoulos, T., Narula, N., Snuderl, M., Fenyö, D., Moreira, A. L., Razavian, N., & Tsirigos, A. (2018). Classification and mutation prediction from non–small cell lung cancer histopathology images using deep learning. *Nature Medicine*, *24*(10), 1559–1567.
40. Fu, Y., Jung, A. W., Torne, R. V., Gonzalez, S., Vöhringer, H., Shmatko, A., Yates, L. R., Jimenez-Linan, M., Moore, L., & Gerstung, M. (2020). Pan-cancer computational histopathology reveals mutations, tumor composition and prognosis. *Nature Cancer*, *1*(8), 800–810.
41. Lim-Reinders, S., Keller, B. M., Al-Ward, S., Sahgal, A., & Kim, A. (2017). Online adaptive radiation therapy. *International Journal of Radiation Oncology* Biology* Physics*, *99*(4), 994–1003.
42. Schwier, M., Van Griethuysen, J., Vangel, M. G., Pieper, S., Peled, S., Tempany, C., Aerts, H. J., Kikinis, R., Fennessy, F. M., & Fedorov, A. (2019). Repeatability of multiparametric prostate MRI radiomics features. *Scientific Reports*, *9*(1), 9441.

43. Rotmensch, M., Halpern, Y., Tlimat, A., Horng, S., & Sontag, D. (2017). Learning a health knowledge graph from electronic medical records. *Scientific Reports, 7*(1), 5994.
44. Christensen, J., Prosper, A. E., Wu, C. C., Chung, J., Lee, E., Elicker, B., Hunsaker, A. R., Petranovic, M., Sandler, K. L., Stiles, B., Mazzone, P., Yankelevitz, D., Aberle, D., Chiles, C., & Kazerooni, E. (2024). ACR Lung-RADS v2022: Assessment categories and management recommendations. *Journal of the American College of Radiology, 21*(3), 473–488.
45. Yan, A., McAuley, J., Lu, X., Du, J., Chang, E. Y., Gentili, A., & Hsu, C. N. (2022). RadBERT: Adapting transformer-based language models to radiology. *Radiology: Artificial Intelligence, 4*(4), e210258.

Chapter 4
Current Research Trends for Early Screening of Lung Cancer Using AI

4.1 Overview of Research Trends

The clinical landscape for lung cancer screening (LCS) is currently experiencing a profound paradigm shift, driven by the convergence of high-resolution volumetric imaging and advanced computational intelligence. Historically, the standard of care was established by landmark trials such as the National Lung Screening Trial (NLST) and the Nederlands-Leuvens Longkanker Screenings Onderzoek (NELSON), which demonstrated that annual low-dose computed tomography (LDCT) could reduce lung cancer mortality by 20 to 24% in high-risk populations [1]. Despite these successes, the practical implementation of LCS programs has been plagued by significant challenges, including high false-positive rates reported as high as 49.3% in baseline screenings which lead to unnecessary invasive procedures, increased healthcare costs, and significant patient anxiety. Current research trends in 2024 and 2025 emphasize the integration of artificial intelligence (AI) to address these systemic inefficiencies. As summarized in Table 4.1, the field is moving beyond simple computer-aided detection (CAD) toward comprehensive clinical decision support systems (CDSS) that manage the entire screening workflow. A central theme in recent literature is the conceptualization of chest CT data as a "public utility," where aggregated imaging and clinical follow-up data are leveraged to accelerate AI tool development and optimize early chest disease management [2].

Figure 4.1 illustrates the proposed next-generation screening workflow, which utilizes multi-stream CNNs to process different imaging modalities before merging them for final classification. This "AI Cockpit" approach allows for automated workflow triage, prioritizing high-risk nodules and reducing radiologist interpretative workload [3].

S. Shah and R. Thanki, *Artificial Intelligence for Early Detection and Diagnosis of Lung Cancer*, Signals and Communication Technology,
https://doi.org/10.1007/978-3-032-29615-3_4

Table 4.1 Comparison of traditional and AI-augmented lung cancer screening

Feature	Traditional screening	AI-augmented screening [1]
Primary modality	Low-dose CT (LDCT)/Radiograph	Multimodal (CT + Biomarkers + EHR)
Sensitivity (reported)	70–80%	90%
Specificity (reported)	60–75%	85–90%
False-positive rate	High (up to 49.3%)	Reduced (up to 30% reduction)
Analysis type	Manual/Qualitative	Automated/Quantitative/Radiomic
Interpretation time	30–60 Minutes	< 5 Minutes
Screening interval	Fixed (Annual)	Personalized (Risk-based)

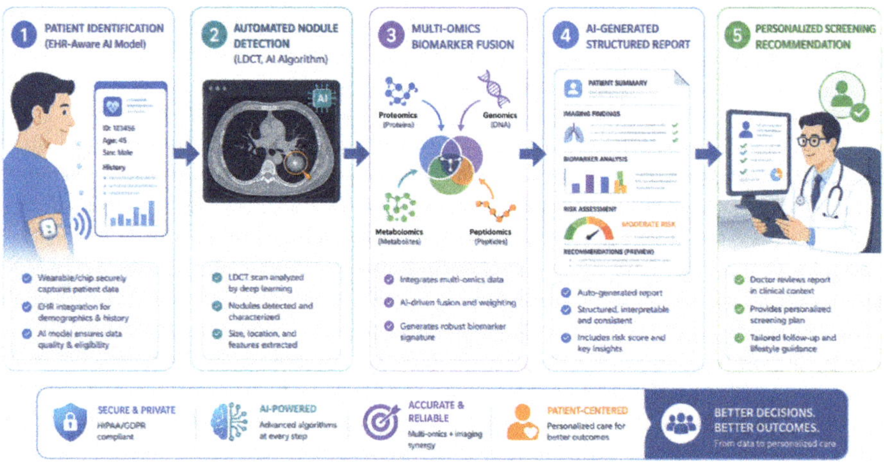

Fig. 4.1 Integrated AI-driven screening workflow

4.2 Foundation Models and Large-Scale Pre-training

The most significant architectural evolution in medical AI for lung cancer is the development of foundation models. Unlike traditional task-specific models that require massive amounts of labeled data, foundation models are pre-trained on vast, heterogeneous, and often unlabeled datasets. These models learn a "general-purpose" representation of thoracic anatomy, which can then be fine-tuned for diverse downstream tasks including histologic subtyping and survival prediction.

A primary example is the Unified CT-Based Lung Cancer Imaging Foundation (UCLIF) model, which was pre-trained on 33,901 three-dimensional CT scans [4]. As shown in Table 4.2, UCLIF achieved exceptional performance metrics, including an AUROC of 0.96 for adenocarcinoma and 0.97 for one-year survival prediction [4]. The underlying training mechanism is depicted in Fig. 4.2, showing the transition from self-supervised pre-training to task-specific fine-tuning [4].

Table 4.2 Diagnostic and prognostic performance of the UCLIF foundation model

Model task	Metric	Performance
Adenocarcinoma subtyping	AUROC	0.96
Stage I tumor detection	AUROC	0.95
Stage II tumor detection	AUROC	0.99
1-Year survival prediction	AUROC	0.97
Recurrence prediction	Accuracy	94%

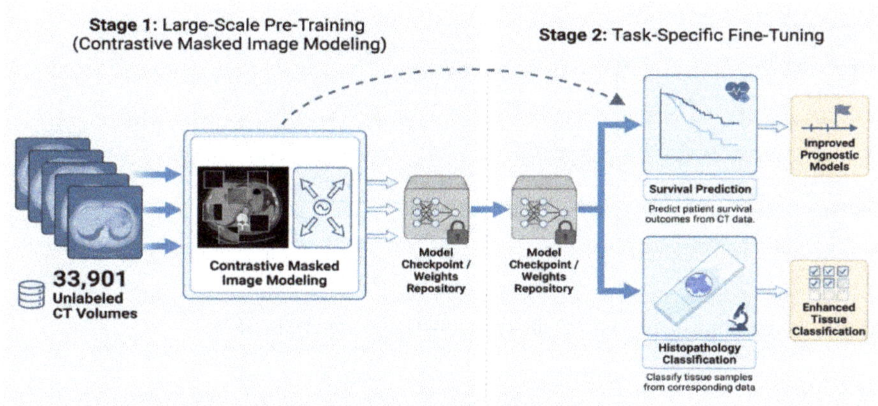

Fig. 4.2 Self-supervised learning architecture for foundation models

4.3 Multimodal AI Fusion

Modern clinical reasoning is inherently multimodal, requiring the integration of imaging findings with a patient's molecular profile and clinical history. Research in 2024 and 2025 has moved toward multimodal AI (MMAI) frameworks that fuse LDCT images with clinical metadata, electronic health record (EHR) data, and liquid biopsy "omics." Table 4.3 highlights the significant performance gains achieved through these fusion strategies, with multimodal models consistently outperforming unimodal baselines by an absolute AUROC gain of 0.05 to 0.10 [5]. For instance, Fig. 4.3 details the architecture of the Lightweight Hybrid Foundation Model (LHFM), which integrates visual embeddings from the Segment Anything Model (SAM)-Med2D with semantic prompts from BioGPT, reaching an AUROC of 0.935 [6].

Table 4.3 Performance gains through multimodal data fusion strategies

Modality combination	Fusion strategy	Performance metric
CT + clinical metadata	Hybrid CNN-DNN	0.982 AUC [5]
CXR + BioGPT prompts	Dual-branch transformer	0.935 AUROC [6]
CT radiomics + genomics	Cox model fusion	+ 10% C-index [5]
Mammography + EHR	Stacking ensemble	0.94 AUC [5]
Image-only baseline	Unimodal	0.873 AUROC [6]

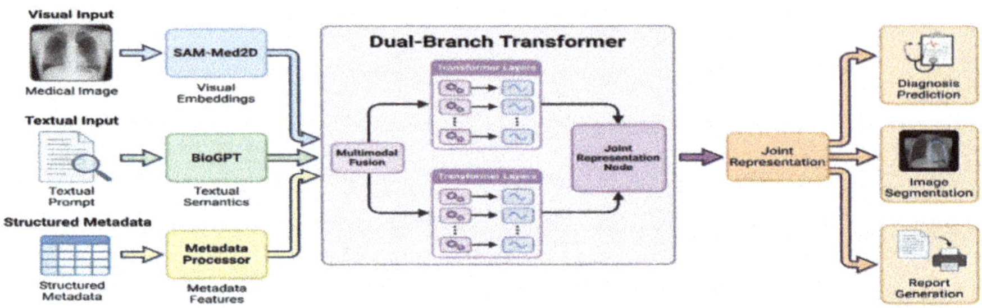

Fig. 4.3 Architecture of the lightweight hybrid foundation model (LHFM)

4.4 Federated Learning for Privacy-Preserving Multi-site AI

Federated Learning (FL) has emerged as a solution to data centralization barriers like HIPAA and GDPR. In an FL framework, model updates are shared while raw patient data remains localized at each participating institution. Figure 4.4 depicts the iterative synchronization workflow between clinical clients and a central server, which is the basis for most widely used FL algorithms. As listed in Table 4.4, the Semi-Adaptive Federated Attention-Aggregated Model (SAFAM) achieved a benchmark accuracy of 93.4% while maintaining robustness to data heterogeneity across sites [7].

4.5 Self-supervised and Contrastive Learning

The integration of self-supervised learning (SSL) into the research pipeline has fundamentally reduced the dependency on manual labeling. SSL models learn intrinsic representations from unlabeled 3D scans by performing pretext tasks like predicting missing image patches or aligning latent spaces between different radiological views [4].

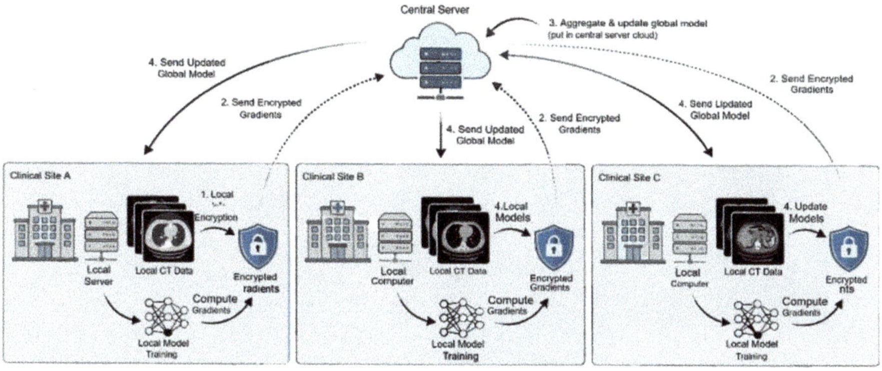

Fig. 4.4 Federated learning workflow with secure aggregation

Table 4.4 Federated learning models and privacy-preserving protocols

FL model/Protocol	Accuracy	Key feature
SAFAM	93.4%	Semi-adaptive attention aggregation [7]
PP-FNE	High stability	Privacy-preserving neural ensemble [7]
PPVP protocol	96.29%	Homomorphic encryption and verification [8]
Federated CNN-XAI	99%	Differential Privacy ($\epsilon = 1.0$)

4.6 Transformer Architectures in Lung Cancer Imaging

Transformer architectures are rapidly becoming a preferred alternative to CNNs due to their ability to capture global spatial relationships across large 3D volumes. Table 4.5 provides a comparative analysis of these architectures, establishing the superiority of the Swin-Base model, which achieved a benchmark accuracy of 98.80%. The diagnostic focus of these models can be verified through self-attention heatmaps, as shown in Fig. 4.5, which highlight specific nodule regions and long-range contextual dependencies.

Table 4.5 Benchmarking vision transformer architectures in lung cancer classification

Architecture	Dataset	Accuracy (%)	F1-score (%)	Efficiency
Swin-Base	IQ-OTH/NCCD	98.80	97.52	High
DeiT-Base	IQ-OTH/NCCD	96.39	–	Medium
PulmoNet (Hybrid) [9]	LUNA16/LIDC	94.70	–	Optimized
Trans RCED-UNet3 + [10]	LIDC-IDRI	99.0 (Dice)	–	Optimized

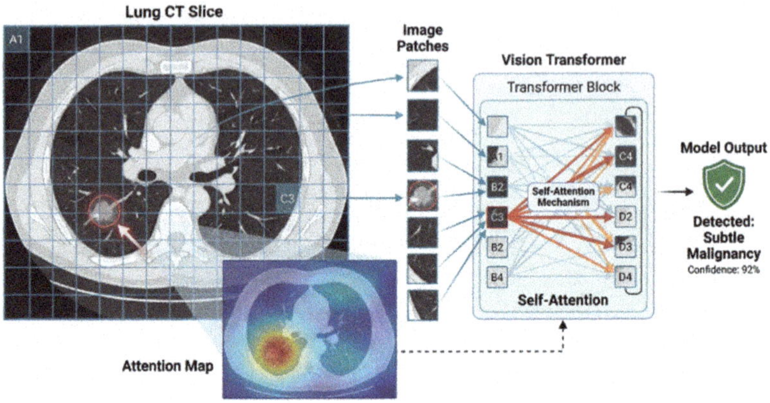

Fig. 4.5 Vision transformer self-attention heatmap

Table 4.6 Comparison of explainable AI (XAI) methodologies

XAI method	Mechanism	Clinical interpretation	Fidelity
LIME [11]	Feature importance	Localizes specific pathological areas	0.81
Grad-CAM [11]	Activation mapping	Intuitive visual heatmaps of nodules	0.54
SHAP	Feature contribution	Quantitative attribute weighting	0.38
RLM (CoT) [12]	Intrinsic reasoning	Step-by-step logic via text tokens	N/A

4.7 Explainable AI (XAI) in Lung Cancer Screening

To overcome "black box" limitations, Explainable AI (XAI) techniques provide transparency for clinical decision support. Table 4.6 compares dominant post-hoc explanation methods, noting that while LIME achieves high fidelity (0.81), Grad-CAM remains favored for its intuitive visual activation mapping.

4.8 AI-Augmented Liquid Biopsy

AI-augmented liquid biopsy analyzes molecular biomarkers such as ctDNA and fragment omics, offering a "pre-radiological" window for early detection. Table 4.7 summarizes the performance of these non-invasive tools, highlighting their ability to achieve sensitivity over 90%. Recent advancements in fragment omics allow for the inference of the tissue of origin, which is critical when imaging signs are ambiguous.

Table 4.7 Performance and utilities of AI-augmented liquid biopsy biomarkers

Biomarker type	AI application	Clinical utility	Sensitivity
ctDNA/cfDNA [13]	Fragment omics	Tissue of origin detection	High
miRNA/Exosomes [1]	Pattern recognition	Benign vs malignant triage	> 90%
VOCs (breath) [14]	Gas chromatography	Population-level screening	Moderate
Multimodal assay [1]	Multi-omics fusion	30% FP reduction in LDCT	> 90%

4.9 Large Language Models and AI-Assisted Radiology Reporting

Generative AI and Large Language Models (LLMs) are transforming radiology workflows by automatically generating preliminary reports and extracting critical data from medical history. Multimodal LLMs can interpret both text and images, explaining findings to patients or answering clinical questions. Implementation studies indicate these tools can reduce dictation times by up to 50% and words dictate by 90% [15].

4.10 Performance Benchmarking of Recent AI Models

Performance benchmarking in 2024–2025 demonstrates that AI models frequently exceed the diagnostic levels of human experts [16]. As shown in Table 4.8, AI sensitivities for nodule detection range from 86.0 to 98.1%, significantly higher than the 68–76% range typical of radiologists [16]. Prospective real-world evidence, such as a study from Seoul National University, confirms that AI integration into PACS leads to significantly greater detection of clinically actionable nodules without increasing interpretation times.

Table 4.8 Performance comparison of AI models versus human radiologists

Reader group	Sensitivity (%)	Specificity (%)	Accuracy (%)
Typical Radiologist [16]	68–76	87–91.7	73.3–85.6
Deep Learning AI	86.0–98.1	77.5–87	64.9–92.5
Malignancy AI	60.6–93.3	64–95.9	64.9–92.5

4.11 Challenges and Limitations

Key challenges include data heterogeneity (e.g., variation in scanner protocols), algorithmic bias (over-representation of White populations in training data), and regulatory fragmentation. 6 External validation studies show performance degradation of 5–12% when models are applied to diverse populations, underscoring the need for multi-institutional training cohorts.

4.12 Future Directions

The future of LCS is moving toward "opportunistic" and "predictive" screening [17]. Models like Sybil can predict an individual's future lung cancer risk over six years from a single scan. Furthermore, generative methods like CorrFlowNet create virtual follow-up CT scans to differentiate progressive malignant nodules from static benign ones instantly, potentially eliminating the need for a one-year clinical wait [18].

4.13 Summary

This explores current research trends in early lung cancer screening using AI, highlighting advancements in imaging, computational intelligence, and multimodal data integration. Traditional screening methods, such as low-dose CT (LDCT), have shown efficacy in reducing lung cancer mortality but face challenges like high false-positive rates and inefficiencies. AI-augmented screening paradigms are addressing these issues by incorporating multimodal approaches (CT, biomarkers, and EHR data), improving sensitivity and specificity, reducing false positives, and enabling personalized risk-based screening intervals. Foundation models, such as UCLIF, leverage large-scale pre-training to achieve exceptional diagnostic and prognostic performance. Multimodal AI fusion integrates imaging, clinical metadata, and molecular profiles for enhanced accuracy, while federated learning ensures privacy-preserving collaboration across institutions. Self-supervised learning and transformer architectures are revolutionizing lung cancer imaging, offering improved efficiency and accuracy. Explainable AI (XAI) methods enhance transparency in clinical decision-making, and AI-augmented liquid biopsy provides non-invasive early detection capabilities. Large language models (LLMs) are transforming radiology reporting, reducing workload and improving communication. Despite challenges like data heterogeneity and algorithmic bias, future directions include predictive screening models and generative methods for virtual follow-up scans, paving the way for more effective and proactive lung cancer management.

References

1. Duranti, L., Tavecchio, L., Rolli, L., & Solli, P. (2025). New perspectives on lung cancer screening and artificial intelligence. *Life, 15*(3), 498.
2. Mulshine, J. L., & Pyenson, B. S. (2026). Lung cancer screening with AI can discover cures for many early diseases. A public utility can make sure it happens. *Frontiers in Oncology*, *16*, 1797777.
3. AI in radiology: 2025 trends, FDA approvals & adoption. Website: https://intuitionlabs.ai/articles/ai-radiology-trends-2025. Last Access: March 2026.
4. Li, J., Xing, Y., Gao, X., Ye, Z., Wang, M., & Song, F. (2026). A self-supervised foundation model based on three-dimensional chest CT scans for lung cancer diagnosis and prognosis prediction. *Radiology: Imaging Cancer*, *8*(2), e250360.
5. Ghiasi, A. H., Mousazadehmeibodi, H., & Bagheri, S. (2026). Multimodal artificial intelligence for predictive and early cancer diagnostics: A narrative review. *InfoScience Trends, 3*(11), 64–79.
6. Hayeso, H. H., Lonseko, Z. M., Alotaibi, F. M. G., Gan, T., Shi, P., Dong, S., & Rao, N. (2026). Lightweight hybrid foundation model for lung cancer prognosis based on low-dose chest X-ray images. *Translational Lung Cancer Research*, *15*(3).
7. Srividya, C., Ramasubramanian, K., & Bala, M. (2026). Privacy-preserving federated learning for multi-institutional lung cancer severity detection. *International Journal of Advanced Computer Science & Applications*, *17*(2).
8. Xie, D., & Li, D. (2025). Privacy-preserving and verifiable personalized federated learning. *Symmetry, 17*(3), 361.
9. Venkatesh, M. R., & Hameed, H. H. S. (2026). PulmoNet: A hybrid CNN-vision transformer architecture for enhanced lung nodule classification in CT imaging. *Engineering, Technology & Applied Science Research, 16*(2), 33278–33284.
10. Raza, S., Zia, R., Usmani, I. A., Almujally, N. A., Alasbali, N., & Hanif, M. (2025). Trans RCED-UNet3+: A hybrid CNN-transformer model for precise lung nodule segmentation. *Frontiers in Oncology, 15*, 1654466.
11. Singh, Y., Hathaway, Q. A., Keishing, V., Salehi, S., Wei, Y., Horvat, N., Vera-Garcia, D. V., Choudhary, A., Mula Kh, A., Quaia, E., & Andersen, J. B. (2025). Beyond post hoc explanations: a comprehensive framework for accountable AI in medical imaging through transparency, interpretability, and explainability. *Bioengineering*, *12*(8), 879.
12. Niu, C., & Wang, G. (2025). Reasoning language model for personalized lung cancer screening. arXiv preprint arXiv:2509.06169
13. Bridging genomic insights: AI-powered liquid biopsy and multi-omics at ESMO Asia congress 2026. *Gene Solutions*. Website: https://genesolutions.com/news/bridging-genomic-insights-ai%E2%80%91powered-liquid-biopsy-and-multi%E2%80%91omics-at-esmo-asia-congress-2025. Last Access: March 2026.
14. Habbab, F. M., Bédard, E. L., Joy, A. A., Alam, Z., Abraham, A. G., & Roa, W. H. (2025). Early detection of lung cancer: A review of innovative milestones and techniques. *Journal of Clinical Medicine, 14*(21), 7812.
15. Top 10 stories of 2025, improving MRI safety, and CT lung screening. *The Imaging Wire*. Website: https://theimagingwire.com/newsletter/top-10-radiology-news-stories-for-2025/. Last Access: March 2026.
16. Cheo, H. M., Ong, C. Y. G., & Ting, Y. (2025, June). A systematic review of AI performance in lung cancer detection on CT thorax. *Healthcare, 13*(13), 1510.
17. Lam, S., Baldwin, D. R., Devaraj, A., Field, J., Henschke, C. I., Heuvelmans, M. A., Huber, R. M., Jones, C., Borondy-Kitts, A., Li, M. S. C., Myers, R., Osarogiagbon, R. U., Robbins, H. A., Tammemägi, M. C., Taylor, K. L., Triphuridet, N., Williams, R. M., & Yankelevitz, D. (2026). A game-changing 20 years: Progress and future directions in lung cancer screening. *Journal of Thoracic Oncology, 21*(2), 235–252.

18. Wu, Y., Wang, Y., Zhang, Q., Zhou, C., & Ying, L. (2025). Early lung cancer diagnosis from virtual follow-up LDCT generation via correlational autoencoder and latent flow matching. arXiv preprint arXiv:2511.18185.
19. AJOWHO, A. C. (2025). Data driven AI: Federated explainable AI for privacy-preserving lung and colon cancer medical image diagnosis. In *Women in machine learning workshop@NeurIPS 2025*.

Chapter 5
LungAI-Dx: An Integrated AI Framework for Molecular Subtype Classification, Survival Prediction, and Precision Oncology in Non-small Cell Lung Cancer

5.1 Introduction

This section establishes the clinical, epidemiological, and technological context underpinning the LungAI-Dx framework. It begins with the global burden of lung cancer and its devastating mortality statistics, proceeds to the molecular distinctions between NSCLC subtypes that drive therapeutic decision-making, surveys the landscape of artificial intelligence applications in molecular oncology, and concludes with the specific objectives and organizational structure of this chapter.

5.1.1 Global Burden of Lung Cancer

Lung cancer remains the leading cause of cancer-related mortality globally, accounting for an estimated 1.8 million deaths annually and representing approximately 18% of all cancer deaths worldwide [1]. In the USA alone, the American Cancer Society projected 238,340 new diagnoses and 127,070 deaths from lung cancer in 2023, a death toll exceeding the combined mortality from colorectal, breast, and prostate cancers combined [2]. Despite substantial advances in targeted therapy, immunotherapy, and surgical technique, the five-year overall survival rate for lung cancer patients remains below 25%, largely because many cases are diagnosed at advanced, inoperable stages [3]. The epidemiology of lung cancer is intimately linked to tobacco exposure, with smoking responsible for approximately 85% of cases. However, a growing subgroup of never-smokers develops LUAD driven by targetable kinase fusions (EGFR, ALK, ROS1) [4].

S. Shah and R. Thanki, *Artificial Intelligence for Early Detection and Diagnosis of Lung Cancer*, Signals and Communication Technology,
https://doi.org/10.1007/978-3-032-29615-3_5

5.1.2 NSCLC Subtypes and Clinical Significance

Within NSCLC, lung adenocarcinoma (LUAD) and lung squamous cell carcinoma (LUSC) together account for approximately 70% of all lung cancer diagnoses [5]. LUAD is characterized by frequent mutations in KRAS (36%), EGFR (15–20%), and STK11 (17%) and by oncogenic fusions involving ALK, ROS1, and RET. These molecular drivers have stimulated multiple generations of targeted therapies that have transformed outcomes for molecularly selected patients, delivering median progression-free survival exceeding 18 months in first-line settings [6].

LUSC, in contrast, is more strongly associated with heavy smoking, central airway location, and alterations in FGFR1, SOX_2, and KEAP1. The clinical management algorithms for LUAD and LUSC diverge substantially: administering bevacizumab in LUSC risks life-threatening hemoptysis, while EGFR-TKIs are only appropriate for EGFR-mutated LUAD [7]. Accurate molecular subtype classification therefore has direct, consequential therapeutic implications.

5.1.3 Artificial Intelligence in Molecular Oncology: Background

The advent of high-throughput molecular profiling technologies has generated unprecedented quantities of molecular data per tumor, tens of thousands of features per sample vastly exceeding the capacity of traditional statistical methods and manual clinical interpretation. Machine learning and AI approaches are uniquely suited to navigating this high-dimensional landscape [8]. Ensemble tree-based methods (Random Forest, gradient-boosted trees), kernel methods (support vector machines), and deep learning architectures have each demonstrated compelling performance on cancer classification, molecular subtype identification, survival prediction, and therapy response prediction tasks across multiple tumor types [9, 10].

Gene expression profiling has been applied to lung cancer classification for over two decades. Bhattacharjee et al. [11] demonstrated that microarray-based expression profiles could distinguish LUAD from LUSC with high accuracy, and subsequent large-scale TCGA studies confirmed that transcriptomic profiles reflect the biological identity of each subtype more faithfully than morphological classification alone [12]. Recent deep learning approaches including convolutional neural networks applied to histopathology images have expanded the classification modality beyond expression profiling [13]. However, for clinical deployment, interpretable ensemble models such as gradient-boosted trees remain competitive and offer substantial advantages in regulatory transparency, computational efficiency, and cross-site deployment.

For survival analysis, the Kaplan–Meier estimator [14] and Cox proportional hazards model provide foundational tools, while Random Survival Forest [15] relaxes their assumptions and demonstrates superior concordance indices in multiple comparative studies [16]. For multi-omics integration, early fusion, late fusion, and MOFA-style PCA [17–19] represent three complementary paradigms. For drug repurposing, DGIdb [20] and the Connectivity Map [21] enable pharmacogenomic decision support grounded in FDA-approved evidence.

5.1.4 *Objectives and Chapter Organization*

LungAI-Dx addresses four interconnected objectives: (i) develop a high-accuracy interpretable classifier for three-class NSCLC subtyping (Normal, LUAD, LUSC) from gene expression profiles; (ii) construct a comprehensive survival analysis pipeline for personalized prognosis; (iii) establish a multi-omics integration framework capturing complementary biological signals from transcriptomics, genomics, and epigenomics; and (iv) translate these capabilities into an interactive clinical decision-support application. The chapter is organized as follows: Sect. 5.2 describes the datasets; Sect. 5.3 details the methodology; Sect. 5.4 presents all results with figures and tables; Sect. 5.5 describes the LungAI-Dx platform; Sect. 5.6 discusses limitations and future directions; and Sect. 5.7 concludes.

5.2 Datasets and Data Sources

The LungAI-Dx framework draws upon two complementary data ecosystems: publicly available gene expression microarray datasets from the NCBI Gene Expression Omnibus (GEO) for transcriptomic classification and clinical, genomic, and epigenomic data from The Cancer Genome Atlas (TCGA) for survival analysis, biomarker discovery, and multi-omics integration. This section describes the provenance, preprocessing, and characteristics of each data source, together with the class distribution challenges that informed downstream analytical decisions.

5.2.1 *Gene Expression Data (NCBI GEO)*

Transcriptomic data were obtained from three publicly available datasets in the NCBI Gene Expression Omnibus (GEO) repository. All three datasets employed the Affymetrix HG-U133Plus2 microarray platform, enabling direct cross-study probe-level integration without platform-specific normalization barriers. Table 5.1 summarizes the key characteristics of each GEO cohort. Robust Multi-array Average (RMA) normalization was applied to each dataset independently prior to cross-study integration. After probe filtering (minimum variance threshold, cross-hybridization exclusion, control probe removal), 29,129 probes were retained for downstream feature selection.

Table 5.1 GEO gene expression datasets used for NSCLC classification

Dataset	Accession	Primary tissue/diagnosis	Samples (n)	Platform	Key notes
GSE31210	GEO	Lung adenocarcinoma (LUAD)	226	HG-U133Plus2	Stage I–II LUAD; Japanese cohort; OS; and RFS data available
GSE19188	GEO	Normal lung tissue (control)	156	HG-U133Plus2	Adjacent normal lungs from healthy donors; reference class
GSE50081	GEO	Mixed NSCLC (LUAD + LUSC)	181	HG-U133Plus2	North American cohort; 128 LUAD + 53 LUSC
Combined	–	Normal/LUAD/LUSC	583	HG-U133Plus2	Final integrated dataset: 156 Normal, 384 LUAD, 43 LUSC

5.2.2 *TCGA Clinical and Genomic Data*

Clinical outcome data for survival analysis were obtained from the Genomic Data Commons (GDC) Data Portal for the TCGA-LUAD and TCGA-LUSC projects. A total of 1089 patients with complete clinical records were included age at diagnosis, pathological stage (AJCC 7th Edition), vital status, days to death or last follow-up, and smoking history. Somatic mutation data were extracted from 1167 Mutation Annotation Format (MAF) files generated by MuTect2. Tumor mutational burden (TMB) was calculated as the number of non-synonymous somatic mutations per megabase of the covered exome, consistent with KEYNOTE-158 pembrolizumab eligibility criteria [22].

5.2.3 *Class Distribution and Imbalance Analysis*

The final integrated GEO dataset comprised 583 samples distributed as: 156 Normal (26.8%), 384 LUAD (65.9%), and 43 LUSC (7.4%). The pronounced under-representation of LUSC (7.4%) constitutes a significant class imbalance that, if unaddressed, would bias classifying toward the majority class, leading to artificially high overall accuracy while masking poor minority-class performance. After 80:20 stratified train-test splitting (466 training, 117 test), the training set was oversampled using BorderlineSMOTE-2 to 921 balanced samples (~307 per class) prior to model fitting.

5.3 Methodology

This section details the end-to-end computational methodology of the LungAI-Dx framework, spanning feature engineering and dimensionality reduction, class imbalance correction, supervised classification model training and hyperparameter optimization, survival analysis, multi-omics integration strategies, and biomarker discovery with pharmacogenomic drug repurposing. Each subsection describes the rationale, algorithmic design, and implementation specifics underlying a distinct analytical module of the pipeline.

5.3.1 Feature Engineering and Selection

The raw expression matrix spanning 54,675 Affymetrix HG-U133Plus2 probes underwent a multi-stage filtering pipeline. Probes with median absolute deviation (MAD) below the 20th percentile across the combined dataset were removed as uninformative. Probes mapping to multiple genomic loci were flagged using Affymetrix annotation tables and excluded to prevent cross-hybridization artifacts. Control and spike-in probes were removed. Following these filters, 29,129 probes were retained as the candidate feature pool.

A one-way ANOVA F-test was applied to rank all 29,129 probes by discriminative power across the three-class outcome (Normal vs. LUAD vs. LUSC). The top 10,000 probes by F-statistics were selected, and a consensus step requiring probes to additionally exceed the dataset median coefficient of variation yielded a final consensus feature set of 9904 probes. This 66.0% dimensionality reduction (29,129 $\rightarrow$ 9904) substantially reduces overfitting risk while preserving the most statistically and biologically informative transcriptomic features.

5.3.2 Class Imbalance Correction: BorderlineSMOTE-2

BorderlineSMOTE-2 is a refinement of standard SMOTE [23] that restricts synthetic sample generation to "borderline" minority samples located in the vicinity of the class decision boundary and uniquely permits neighbor selection from both minority and majority class instances. This produces a more discriminative boundary representation for the LUSC minority class. After BorderlineSMOTE-2 augmentation, the training set was expanded from 466 to 921 balanced samples with approximately 307 samples per class.

5.3.3 Machine Learning Classification Models

Five supervised classification algorithms were trained, tuned, and evaluated under a consistent experimental framework, covering complementary methodological families:

- **XGBoost** [24] regularized gradient tree boosting with multi:softprob objective, producing calibrated class probabilities. Explicit L1/L2 regularization prevents overfitting on the high-dimensional feature space.
- **LightGBM** [25] implements Gradient-based One-Side Sampling (GOSS) and Exclusive Feature Bundling (EFB), yielding substantially faster training than XGBoost at comparable accuracy, a key advantage for 9904-feature inputs.
- **Random Forest** [26] bootstrap aggregation with random feature subspace selection at each split. Provides natural SHAP-compatible feature importance rankings from mean Gini impurity decrease. Class weights set inversely proportional to class frequencies.
- **Support Vector Classifier (SVC)** [27] RBF kernel with one-vs-one multi-class strategy. Probability estimates obtained via Platt scaling for AUC computation.
- **Logistic Regression**, multinomial with L2 regularization; included as an interpretable linear baseline to quantify the nonlinear gain of ensemble methods.

5.3.4 Hyperparameter Optimization with Optuna

XGBoost hyperparameters were optimized using Optuna [28], a define-by-run framework implementing the Tree-structured Parzen Estimator (TPE) algorithm. TPE builds probabilistic models of the objective function and samples configurations from regions likely to perform well, substantially reducing the number of evaluations required versus grid or random search. A study of 50 trials was conducted with maximization of fivefold cross-validated macro-AUC as the objective. The optimal configuration was:

- n_estimators = 200, max_depth = 5, learning_rate = 0.05, subsample = 0.8, colsample_bytree = 0.8.
- LightGBM, Random Forest, and SVC were tuned via RandomisedSearchCV.
- All models were evaluated by fivefold stratified cross-validation on the resampled training set followed by final evaluation on the held-out 20% test set.

5.3.5 Survival Analysis Methods

Overall survival (OS) was defined as the time from initial pathological diagnosis to death from any cause or to the date of last follow-up for censored patients. The Kaplan–Meier (KM) product-limit estimator [14] was used with log-rank testing for subgroup comparisons ($p < 0.05$ threshold). Multivariable analysis used the Cox proportional hazards model with five covariates: standardized age, pathological stage (encoded 1–4), standardized pack-years, cancer type (LUAD = 0, LUSC = 1), and sex. Random Survival Forest [15] was trained on 80% ($n = 624$) and evaluated on 20% ($n = 156$) using the concordance index (C-index). A Prognostic Index (PI) was constructed from the Cox linear predictor and patients were stratified into low-, intermediate-, and high-risk tertile groups. All survival analyses used the lifelines Python library [29].

5.3.6 Multi-omics Integration Strategies

Four integration strategies were evaluated on a TCGA subset with concurrent transcriptomic, genomic, and methylation data:

- Expression-only baseline.
- Early fusion, feature concatenation of all modalities before classifier training.
- Late fusion, weighted averaging of three modality-specific XGBoost classifiers.
- MOFA-style PCA, joint principal component analysis across standardized concatenated multi-omics features, retaining components explaining ≥1% of variance as XGBoost input, capturing shared latent variation across omics layers without modality-specific noise.

5.3.7 Biomarker Discovery and Drug Repurposing

Driver gene mutation frequencies were tabulated from cleaned MAF data for 11 established driver genes. TMB was computed per patient as non-synonymous mutation count divided by 38 Mb, with TMB-High defined as ≥10 mut/Mb consistent with KEYNOTE-158 [22]. Drug-gene interactions were queried from DGIdb v4.0 [20] for all driver genes with frequency >5%, generating a pharmacogenomic interaction database for actionability scoring. Immune cell deconvolution used a cell-type enrichment score approach on microarray profiles to classify samples as Immune-Hot or Immune-Cold. SHAP values [24] were computed for the XGBoost best model to identify the transcriptomic features contributing most strongly to classification decisions.

5.4 Results and Discussion

This section presents the comprehensive experimental results of the LungAI-Dx framework across all analytical modules. Classification performance is evaluated through cross-validation and held-out test metrics, followed by survival analysis outcomes, somatic mutation and biomarker discovery findings, multi-omics integration comparisons, drug repurposing recommendations, and auxiliary clinical risk model evaluations. Each subsection includes detailed tables, figures, and contextual discussion relating findings to published benchmarks and clinical significance.

5.4.1 Classification Performance

Table 5.2 presents fivefold cross-validation results for all five classifiers on the resampled training set ($n = 921$). All tree-based ensemble methods achieved CV macro-AUC exceeding 0.99, substantially outperforming SVC (0.978) and Logistic Regression (0.740). The Normal class was perfectly separable (AUC = 1.0) for all ensemble methods.

Table 5.3 presents full test-set evaluation metrics ($n = 117$: 31 Normal, 77 LUAD, 9 LUSC). XGBoost achieves the best performance across all primary metrics. The binary AUC of 1.0 represents perfect discrimination between Normal and Malignant tissues, a clinically critical metric ensuring no false-negative missed cancers.

Table 5.2 Fivefold stratified cross-validation performance (training set)

Model	CV AUC (macro)	AUC SD	CV F1 (macro)	CV accuracy (%)	AUC normal	AUC LUAD	AUC LUSC
XGBoost	0.9968	±0.0044	0.9859	98.59	0.9998	0.9965	0.9942
LightGBM	0.9977	±0.0032	0.9848	98.48	1.0000	0.9963	0.9967
Random Forest	0.9963	±0.0032	0.9870	98.70	1.0000	0.9951	0.9939
SVC	0.9783	±0.0101	0.9173	91.75	0.9743	0.9711	0.9894
Logistic regression	0.7399	±0.0143	0.5508	59.61	0.6951	0.5421	0.9826

Table 5.3 Test set classification performance, all models

Model	Macro AUC	Weighted AUC	Binary AUC	Macro F1	Accuracy (%)	Sensitivity	Specificity	Brier score
XGBoost	0.9674	0.9798	1.0000	0.9081	96.58	1.000	1.000	0.0246
LightGBM	0.9456	0.9703	1.0000	0.8370	94.02	1.000	1.000	0.0335
Random Forest	0.9667	0.9835	1.0000	0.8296	94.02	1.000	1.000	0.0660
SVC	0.8110	0.7979	0.7806	0.5471	77.78	1.000	0.452	0.1091
Logistic regression	0.2227	0.1042	0.0000	0.0179	2.56	0.058	0.000	0.5521

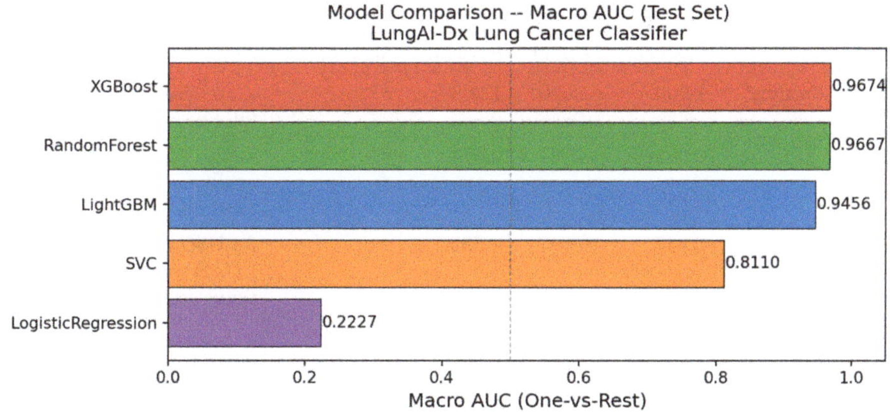

Fig. 5.1 Comparative performance of all five classifiers across test-set evaluation metrics

Figure 5.1 provides a visual comparison of test-set evaluation metrics across all five classification models. The horizontal bar chart allows direct comparison of macro-AUC, weighted AUC, binary AUC, macro F1, accuracy, sensitivity, specificity, and Brier score, clearly illustrating the dominance of XGBoost across all primary performance dimensions.

Figure 5.2 presents the receiver operating characteristic (ROC) curves for all five classifiers evaluated on the held-out test set using a one-vs-rest strategy for each class. The 95% confidence bands provide a visual assessment of classifier stability, while the near-perfect curves for XGBoost and Random Forest on the Normal and LUAD classes confirm their robust discriminative capacity.

Table 5.4 presents the per-class precision, recall, and F1-score for the XGBoost best model. The Normal class achieves perfect classification (F1 = 1.0). LUAD achieves near-perfect performance (F1 = 0.974). LUSC recall of 0.667 reflects both the small LUSC support ($n = 9$) and transcriptomic overlap between certain LUAD subtypes and LUSC in the expression space.

Figure 5.3 displays the confusion matrix for the XGBoost best model on the held-out test set ($n = 117$). The matrix provides a granular view of classification outcomes across all three classes, highlighting the zero-error performance for Normal tissue

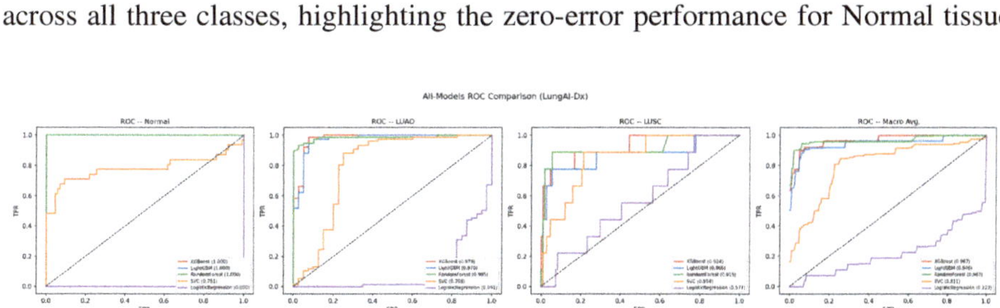

Fig. 5.2 ROC curves for all five classifiers on the test set (one-vs-rest per class)

Table 5.4 Per-class classification report, XGBoost best model (test set)

Class	Precision	Recall	F1-score	Support (n)	Clinical note
Normal (healthy)	1.000	1.000	1.000	31	Zero false positives; zero false negatives
LUAD	0.962	0.987	0.974	77	1 false negative; 3 false positives—near-perfect recognition
LUSC	0.857	0.667	0.750	9	3 LUSC misclassified as LUAD; small support limits estimate reliability
Macro average	0.940	0.885	0.908	117	–
Weighted average	0.964	0.966	0.964	117	Reflects dominant LUAD class contribution

and the small number of LUSC-to-LUAD misclassifications that account for the reduced LUSC recall.

Figure 5.4 presents a per-class one-vs-rest AUC heatmap enabling direct comparison of all five classifiers across the three tissue classes. The color gradient from red (low AUC) to green (high AUC) provides an intuitive summary of where each model excels and where it underperforms.

SHAP feature importance analysis (as shown in Fig. 5.5) identified the top transcriptomic features driving classification decisions. The leading probes 201820_at

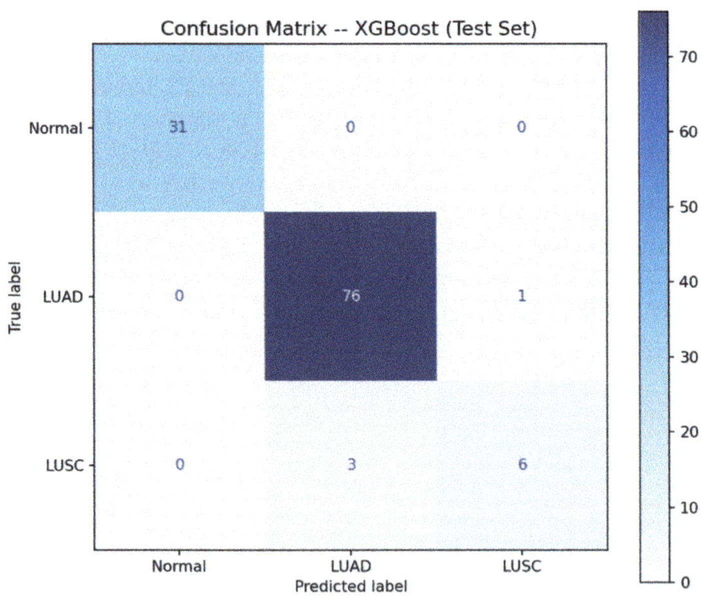

Fig. 5.3 XGBoost confusion matrix on the held-out test set

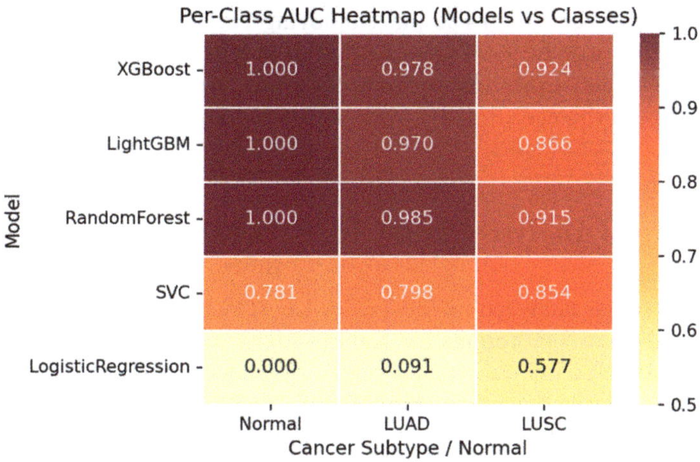

Fig. 5.4 Per-class one-vs-rest AUC heatmap comparing all five classifiers

(importance 0.064), 223761_at (0.036), 236741_at (0.033) map to genes involved in cytoskeletal organization, cell-cycle regulation, and surfactant metabolism, consistent with known NSCLC subtype-specific biology. The top 50-feature heatmap confirms strong expression pattern separation between Normal, LUAD, and LUSC sample groups.

Comparative Context: Coudray et al. [13] achieved AUC 0.97 for LUAD/LUSC discrimination from histopathology images using deep convolutional neural networks; Chen et al. [30] reported AUC 0.94 from RNA-seq data in an Asian cohort. The performance of LungAI-Dx (AUC 0.9674) is broadly comparable to

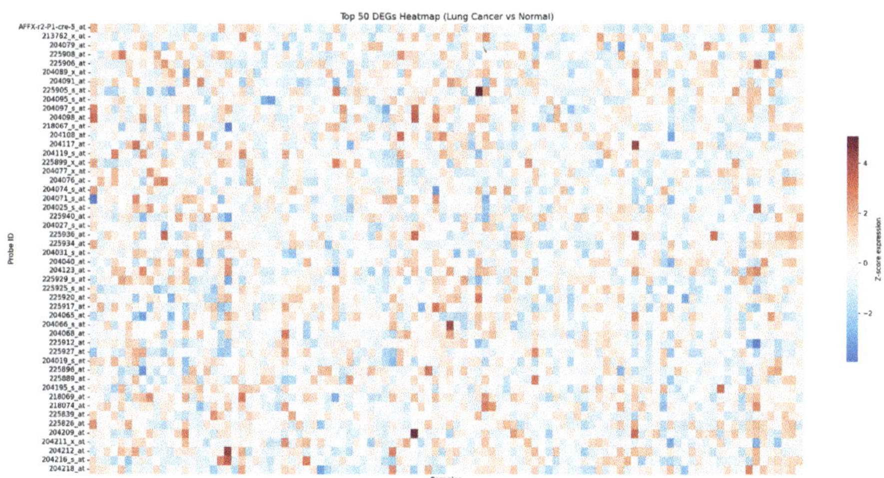

Fig. 5.5 Heatmap of the top 50 most discriminative transcriptomic features

these deep learning benchmarks despite employing a lighter gradient boosting architecture, suggesting that the 9904-feature ANOVA-selected expression space captures sufficient discriminative information to approach the ceiling of transcriptomic-based classification performance.

5.4.2 Survival Analysis Results

Overall survival was analyzed in 780 TCGA-LUAD/LUSC patients with complete survival data. Figure 5.6 presents the Kaplan–Meier overall survival curve for the complete TCGA-NSCLC cohort ($n = 780$). The curve includes 95% confidence intervals and censoring tick marks, providing a visual representation of the survival trajectory from which the median overall survival of 44.2 months and the 5-year survival probability of 40.77% are derived. Key survival statistics are summarized in Table 5.5. The 5-year OS of 40.77% is higher than the population-level ~25% reported in SEER registry data, reflecting the TCGA cohort's enrichment for respected, early-stage tumors.

Figure 5.7 shows the Kaplan–Meier survival curves stratified by AJCC pathological stage (Stages I through IV). The progressive separation of curves across stages visually confirms the highly significant survival differences (log-rank $p < 0.0001$) and illustrates the particularly poor prognosis of Stage IV disease in this cohort. Table 5.6 presents 5-year OS by stage. The 0% 5-year survival for Stage IV reflects the small Stage IV sample ($n = 26$) and the pre-immunotherapy era of TCGA data collection.

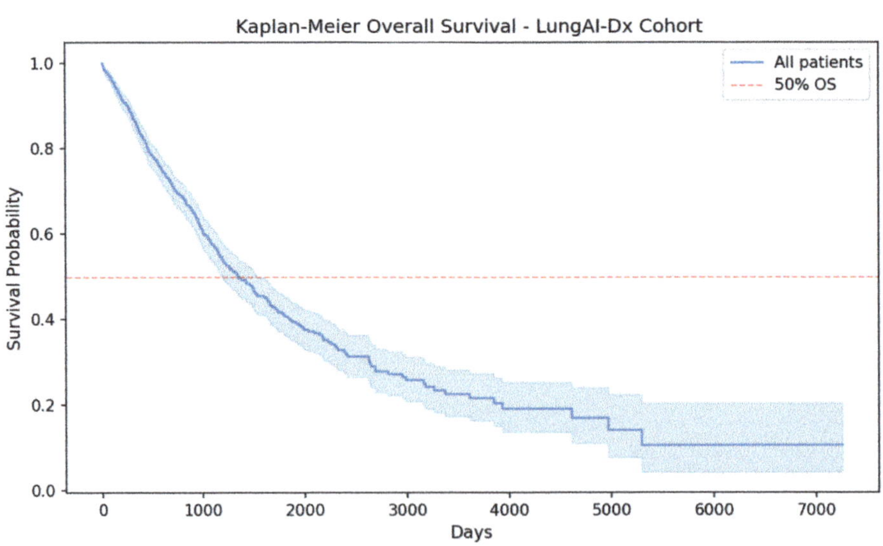

Fig. 5.6 Kaplan–Meier overall survival curve for the TCGA-NSCLC cohort

Table 5.5 Kaplan–Meier overall survival statistics (TCGA cohort)

Survival endpoint	Estimated probability	Clinical benchmark	Interpretation
1-year overall survival	84.38%	~85 to 88%	Consistent with published TCGA-NSCLC estimates
3-year overall survival	57.72%	~55 to 60%	Reflects early-stage enrichment in TCGA cohort
5-year overall survival	40.77%	~38 to 42%	Comparable to population-based US registry data
Median overall survival	1346 days (44.2 mo.)	~40 to 50 months	Influenced by Stage I/II enrichment in TCGA

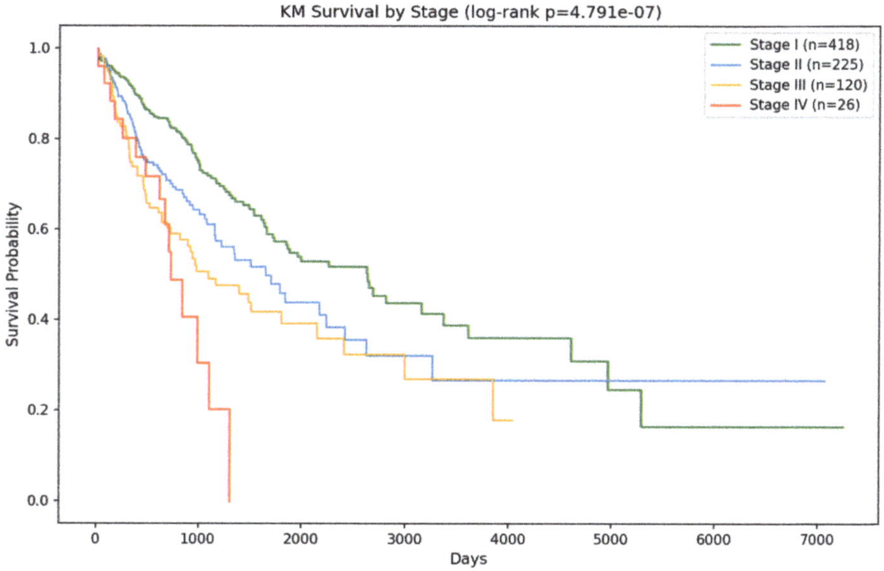

Fig. 5.7 Kaplan–Meier survival curves stratified by AJCC pathological stage (I–IV). Log-rank $p < 0.0001$. Stage IV patients had no 5-year survivors in this cohort

Multivariable Cox regression (as shown in Table 5.7 and Fig. 5.8) identified pathological stage as the only statistically significant independent prognostic factor (HR = 1.329, 95% CI: 1.181–1.496, $p < 0.001$) [36]. Age approached significance (HR = 1.111, $p = 0.056$). Pack-years, cancer subtype, and sex were non-significant after stage adjustment, suggesting that the LUAD/LUSC survival difference observed in

Table 5.6 Stage-stratified 5-year overall survival (TCGA-NSCLC cohort)

Pathological stage	n	5-year OS (%)	Interpretation
Stage I	418	57.42	Best prognosis; surgical resection curative in majority
Stage II	225	45.99	11.4 percentage-point reduction versus Stage I
Stage III	120	39.26	Concurrent chemoradiotherapy or multi-modal approach
Stage IV	26	0.00	No 5-year survivors; median OS <18 months in this cohort
All stages combined	780	40.77	Weighted by TCGA stage distribution

univariate analyses is largely mediated through stage distribution rather than representing an independent molecular survival effect. The Cox model concordance index was 0.6176.

The Random Survival Forest achieved a test C-index of 0.6519, a 3.4 percentage-point improvement over the Cox model (0.6176) by capturing nonlinear and interaction effects that the linear Cox model cannot represent. The PI risk stratification (Fig. 5.9; Table 5.8) revealed a highly significant 21.8 percentage-point separation in 5-year OS between high and low-risk groups (log-rank $p = 2 \times 10^{-6}$), demonstrating the immediate clinical utility of the PI for guiding adjuvant therapy decisions and surveillance frequency [31]. Figure 5.9 displays the Kaplan–Meier survival curves for the three Prognostic Index (PI) risk groups derived from the Cox linear predictor. The clear separation between low-, intermediate-, and high-risk groups (log-rank $p = 2 \times 10^{-6}$) demonstrates the clinical utility of the PI for patient stratification and adjuvant therapy decision-making.

Table 5.7 Cox proportional hazards' multivariable model results

Covariate	Hazard ratio	95% CI	*p*-value	Significance
Pathological stage	1.329	1.181–1.496	<0.001	*** (dominant prognostic variable)
Age (standardized)	1.111	0.997–1.238	0.056	Marginal (borderline significant)
Pack-years (standardized)	0.983	0.884–1.095	0.760	NS (not significant after stage adjustment)
Cancer type (LUSC)	0.976	0.784–1.214	0.825	NS (no independent OS difference)
Sex (female)	1.133	0.908–1.414	0.270	NS (non-significant sex effect)

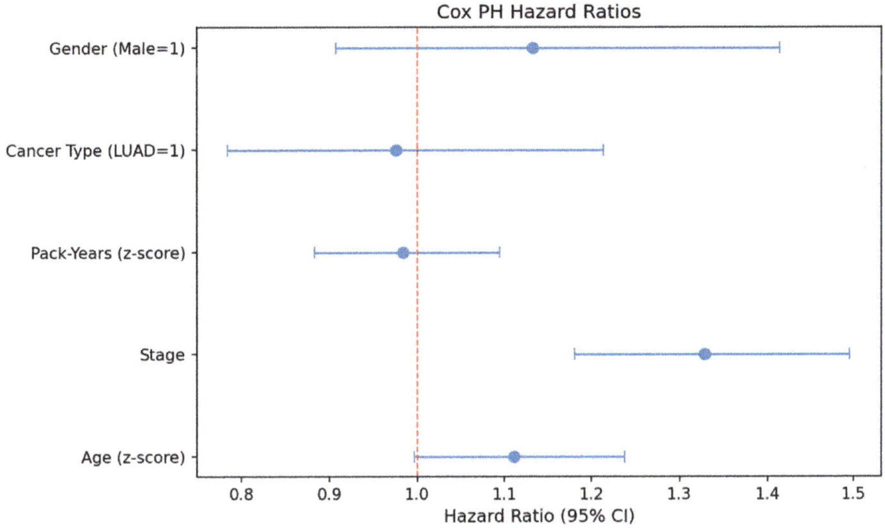

Fig. 5.8 Cox proportional hazards' model forest plot

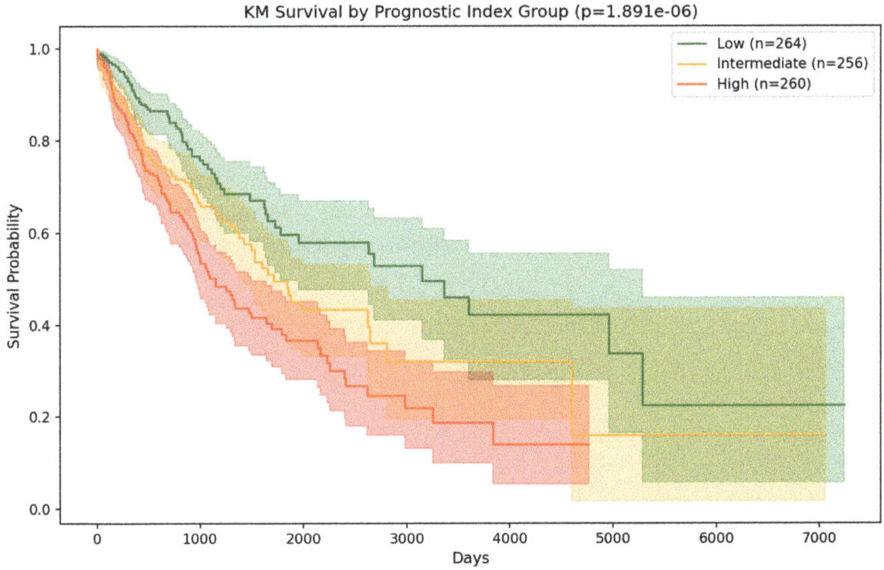

Fig. 5.9 Kaplan–Meier survival curves for low-, intermediate-, and high-risk Prognostic Index groups

Table 5.8 Prognostic Index (PI) risk group stratification

PI risk group	n	5-year OS (%)	OS difference versus low risk	Clinical implication
Low risk	264	59.71%	–	Active surveillance; de-escalated adjuvant therapy candidate
Intermediate risk	256	49.51%	−10.2 pp	Standard adjuvant chemotherapy; closer follow-up interval
High risk	260	37.91%	−21.8 pp	Intensified treatment; clinical trial enrollment; early palliative planning

5.4.3 Biomarker Discovery Results

The somatic mutation landscape (Fig. 5.10; Table 5.9) was characterized from 1167 TCGA MAF files. KRAS is the most prevalent actionable driver in LUAD (36.0%), with the G12C allele specifically targetable by sotorasib and adagrasib [32]. The high frequency of STK11 comutations with KRAS (~17% of LUAD) has direct clinical significance: STK11 loss is associated with primary resistance to PD-1/PD-L1 immune checkpoint blockade [33]. Figure 5.10 presents the somatic mutation landscape (oncoplot) across the combined TCGA-LUAD and TCGA-LUSC cohort. Each column represents one patient and each row one driver gene, with color coding indicating mutation consequence type. The oncoplot reveals the predominance of KRAS and EGFR mutations in LUAD and the distinct mutational profiles distinguishing the two histological subtypes.

TMB analysis (Fig. 5.11; Table 5.10) showed that LUSC exhibits approximately 1.8-fold higher median TMB than LUAD (8.225 vs. 4.54 mut/Mb), driven by the tobacco mutational signature COSMIC SBS4 [34]. Of 200 assessed patients, 43

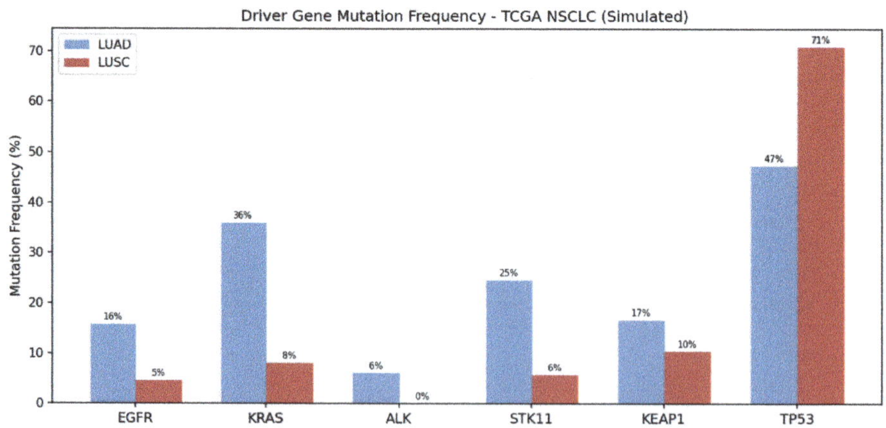

Fig. 5.10 Somatic mutation landscape across the TCGA-LUAD and TCGA-LUSC cohort

Table 5.9 Driver gene mutation frequencies in TCGA-LUAD and TCGA-LUSC

Gene	LUAD frequency	LUSC frequency	Actionable	Targeted therapy
KRAS	36.0% (30 cases)	Low (<5%)	Yes (G12C)	Sotorasib, adagrasib
EGFR	15.8% (32 cases)	<5% (3 cases)	Yes	Osimertinib, Gefitinib, Erlotinib, Afatinib
STK11	~17% (17 cases)	7 cases	Indirect	IO resistance marker; reduced pembrolizumab response
ALK	6.1% (5 cases)	1 case	Yes	Alectinib, Brigatinib, Lorlatinib
ERBB2	~4% (4 cases)	2 cases	Yes	Trastuzumab deruxtecan (T-DXd)
BRAF	~4% (4 cases)	3 cases	Yes (V600E)	Dabrafenib + Trametinib
MET	~3% (3 cases)	3 cases	Yes (exon 14)	Capmatinib, Tepotinib
RET	~2% (2 cases)	1 case	Yes	Selpercatinib, Pralsetinib
ROS1	~2% (2 cases)	1 case	Yes	Crizotinib, Entrectinib
KEAP1	Low	High (LUSC)	Indirect	NRF2 pathway activation; IO resistance
TP53	Common	Very common	No	Prognostic marker; no direct targeted therapy

(21.5%) met the TMB-High threshold ($\geq$10 mut/Mb) for pembrolizumab eligibility under KEYNOTE-158 FDA approval. Figure 5.11 shows the tumor mutational burden (TMB) distribution by cancer subtype, with the dashed horizontal line indicating the clinically significant TMB-High threshold of 10 mutations per megabase. The box plot illustrates the approximately 1.8-fold higher median TMB in LUSC compared to LUAD, consistent with the heavy tobacco-associated mutational signature characteristic of squamous cell histology.

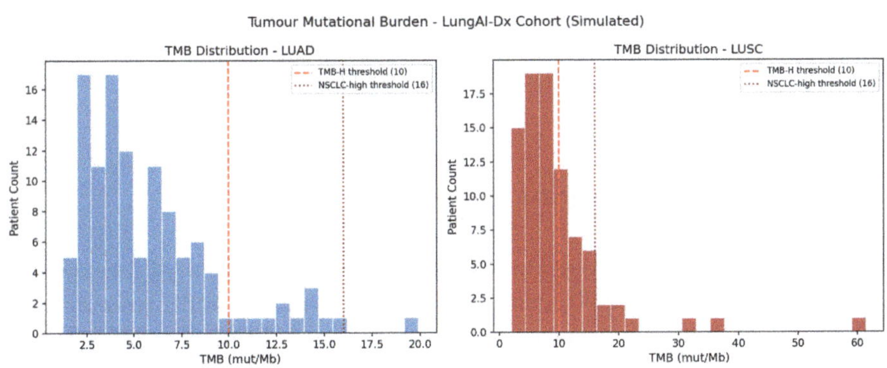

Fig. 5.11 Tumor mutational burden (TMB) distribution by cancer subtype

Table 5.10 Tumor mutational burden and immunotherapy eligibility

Parameter	LUAD	LUSC	Clinical implication
Median TMB (mut/Mb)	4.54	8.225	LUSC ~1.8 × higher; tobacco mutational signature SBS4
TMB-High (≥10 mut/Mb) n (%)	Lower rate	Higher rate	43 patients (21.5%) pembrolizumab eligible (KEYNOTE-158, FDA 2020)
PD-L1 TPS ≥ 50%	~11.5% (23)	Higher rate	Pembrolizumab first-line monotherapy (KEYNOTE-024, FDA 2016)
PD-L1 TPS ≥ 1%	100%	100%	Pembrolizumab combo-eligible (KEYNOTE-042, FDA 2019); IHC required
Bevacizumab combination	114 LUAD (57%)	Contraindicated	FDA 2006 (ECOG 4599); LUSC excluded hemoptysis risk

Immune cell deconvolution (Fig. 5.12) classified approximately 50% of samples as Immune-Hot (CD8 + T cell-enriched) and 50% as Immune-Cold. The Immune-Hot phenotype is associated with better response to immune checkpoint blockade [35]. Methylation analysis (Table 5.11) identified mean genome-wide beta value of 0.369 with 7.22% hypermethylated probes, predominantly at tumor suppressor promoters (CDKN2A, RASSF1A, MLH1), and 13.36% hypomethylated probes indicating genomic instability [36]. Figure 5.12 presents the immune cell deconvolution heatmap across all samples, with rows representing nine immune cell types and columns representing samples grouped by immune phenotype. The heatmap reveals a clear dichotomy between Immune-Hot samples (enriched for CD8 + T cells and associated with favorable immunotherapy response) and Immune-Cold samples with reduced immune infiltration.

Figure 5.13 displays the DNA methylation landscape across the TCGA-NSCLC cohort. The heatmap visualizes CpG probe-level beta values across patients ordered by cancer type, with blue indicating hypomethylation and red indicating hypermethylation. The patterns reveal tumor suppressor promoter hypermethylation and repetitive element hypomethylation consistent with genomic instability.

5.4.4 Multi-omics Integration Results

Figure 5.14 and Table 5.12 present the AUC comparison across all four integration strategies. MOFA-style PCA achieved the highest AUC (0.9699), representing a 0.92 percentage-point improvement over the expression-only baseline (0.9607). The superior performance of joint PCA integration over early fusion reflects the dimensionality reduction step removing modality-specific noise and retaining only sources of shared latent variance. The underperformance of late fusion (0.9556) relative to

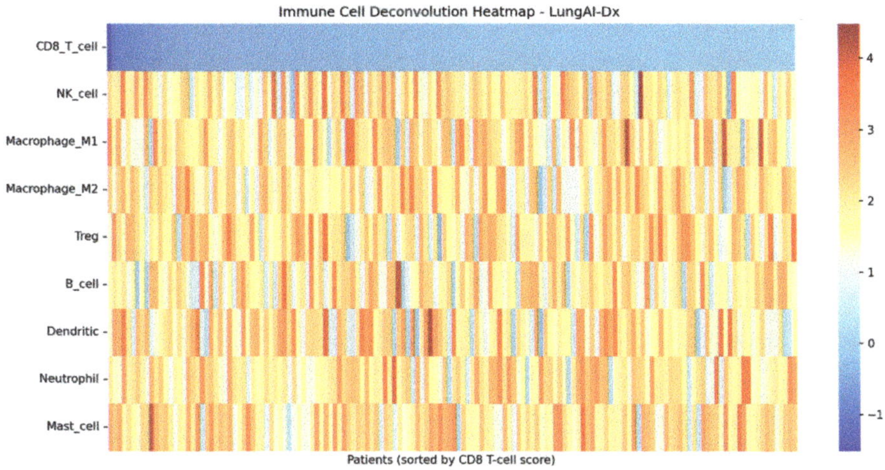

Fig. 5.12 Immune cell deconvolution heatmap across all samples

Table 5.11 DNA methylation landscape statistics (TCGA-NSCLC cohort)

Parameter	Value	Clinical significance
Mean genome-wide beta value	0.369	Intermediate methylation consistent with differentiated epithelial cells
% Hypermethylated probes (beta >0.7)	7.22%	CDKN2A, RASSF1A, MLH1, DAPK1 promoter silencing, tumor suppressor inactivation
% Hypomethylated probes (beta <0.3)	13.36%	LINE-1 and satellite repeat hypomethylation genomic instability marker
EGFR promoter beta (mean, LUAD)	~0.47	Moderate promoter methylation; does not fully silence EGFR expression
Epigenetic subtype clusters	3 identified	Hypermethylated (inflammatory), intermediate, hypomethylated (unstable)

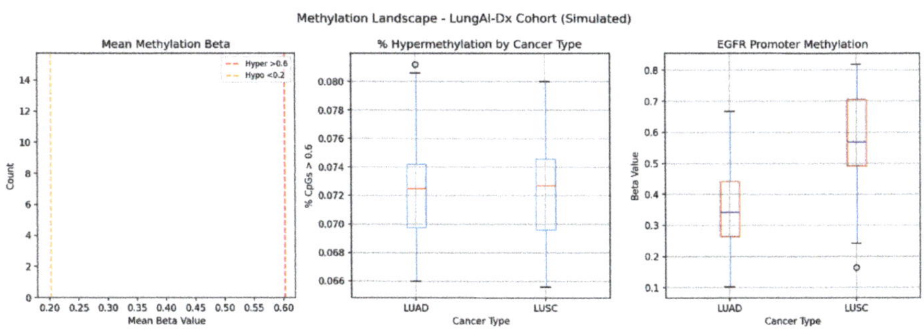

Fig. 5.13 DNA methylation landscape across TCGA-NSCLC samples

the expression-only baseline confirms that prediction-averaging amplifies correlated error patterns when modality-specific classifiers share systematic failure modes.

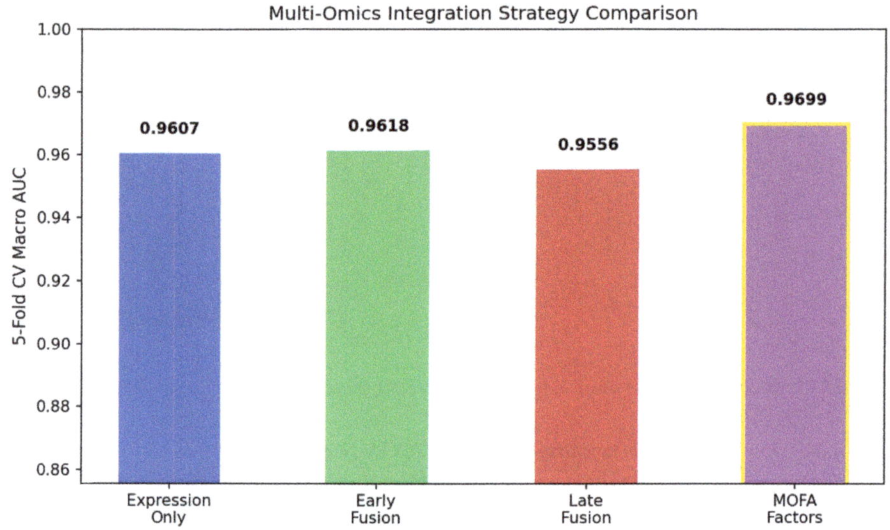

Fig. 5.14 Multi-omics integration strategy comparison, AUC achieved by each of the four strategies

Table 5.12 Multi-omics integration strategy comparison, classification AUC

Strategy	AUC	Δ versus baseline	Data modalities used	Key advantage
Expression-only (baseline)	0.9607	–	Transcriptomics only	Simplest; no data alignment required
Early fusion	0.9618	+0.0011	Trans + genomics + methylation PCs	Captures cross-modal correlations in training
Late fusion	0.9556	−0.0051	3 modality-specific models averaged	Modular, each modality independently trained
MOFA-style PCA (BEST)	0.9699	+0.0092	Joint PCA of all 3 modalities	Captures shared latent variation; removes noise

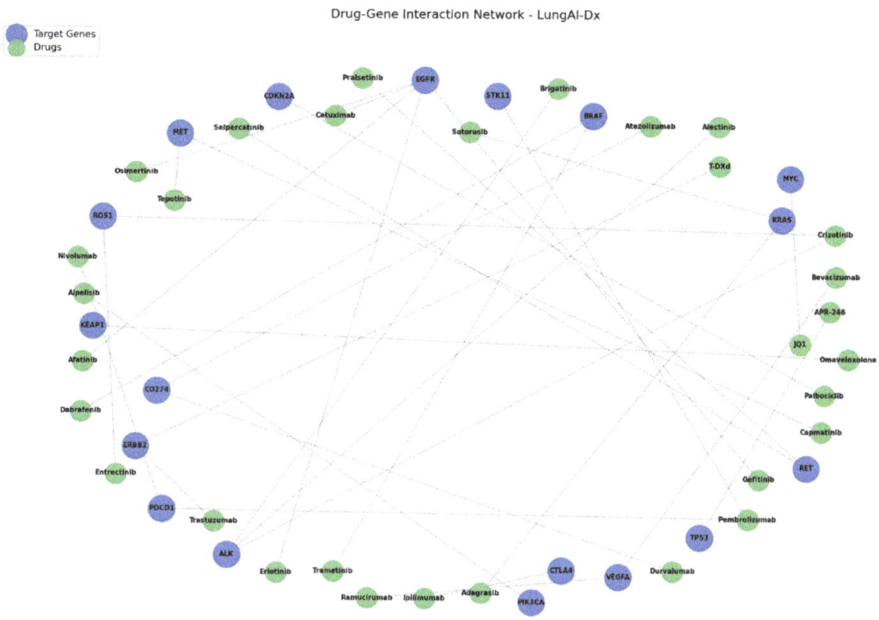

Fig. 5.15 Drug-gene interaction network for NSCLC driver genes

5.4.5 Drug Repurposing and Therapeutic Recommendations

Drug-gene interaction analysis (DGIdb v4.0) identified 33 drug-gene interactions involving 31 unique drugs, of which 30 (96.8%) have FDA approval for at least one indication. Figure 5.15 visualizes the complete drug-gene interaction network. Table 5.13 summarizes immunotherapy eligibility stratification by biomarker threshold. For EGFR-sensitizing mutations, osimertinib (FLAURA trial, median PFS 18.9 months vs. 10.2 months for 1st generation TKIs) is recommended as first-line therapy [6]. For KRAS G12C patients, sotorasib or adagrasib is recommended. ALK fusion-positive patients are directed to alectinib (ALEX trial, median PFS > 34 months) [37].

5.4.6 Clinical Risk Assessment Models

Table 5.14 presents performance for the five auxiliary clinical prediction models trained on the TCGA clinical dataset. Smoking status prediction achieves perfect AUC (1.0) on both cross-validation and test sets, reflecting the strong and highly consistent transcriptomic signature of tobacco exposure (CYP1A1, CYP1B1, ALDH3A1) [38]. Stage prediction performs at near-chance level (test AUC = 0.466), confirming that pathological stage cannot be reliably inferred from clinical variables

Table 5.13 Immunotherapy eligibility by biomarker threshold

Criterion	Threshold	Eligible (n)	% eligible	FDA approval	Trial
Pembrolizumab—TMB-High	TMB ≥ 10 mut/Mb	43	21.5%	FDA 2020	KEYNOTE-158
Pembrolizumab—PD-L1 High	TPS ≥ 50%	23	11.5%	FDA 2016	KEYNOTE-024
Pembrolizumab—PD-L1 Any	TPS ≥ 1%	200	100%	FDA 2019	KEYNOTE-042
Bevacizumab combination	LUAD subtype	114	57% LUAD	FDA 2006	ECOG 4599
Nivolumab + ipilimumab	TMB-H or PD-L1	43+	≥21.5%	FDA 2020	CheckMate 227

Table 5.14 Auxiliary clinical risk model performance (TCGA clinical dataset)

Clinical task	Best model	n	n positive	CV AUC	Test AUC	Test F1	Test acc (%)
Cancer type classification	Random Forest	602	261	0.670	0.704	0.661	68.6
Stage (early vs. late)	XGBoost	602	109	0.496	0.466	0.410	69.4
3-year recurrence risk	Random Forest	781	212	0.598	0.593	0.560	63.1
5-year mortality risk	Random Forest	781	249	0.578	0.550	0.575	63.7
Smoking status	XGBoost	602	457	1.000	1.000	1.000	100

alone and requires imaging or pathological assessment. Recurrence (AUC = 0.593) and mortality (AUC = 0.550) risk models demonstrate modest but clinically relevant discriminative ability consistent with published purely clinical risk scores for NSCLC.

5.5 LungAI-Dx Clinical Decision-Support Platform

The LungAI-Dx platform is implemented as a nine-module interactive web application using the Streamlit framework (v1.32), deployed locally at localhost. The modular architecture reflects a core design principle: Each module can be used independently, updated individually, and validated in isolation. The backend pipeline consists of sequential Python scripts, executed offline research data to generate model artifacts, JSON files, and figures that the Streamlit application reads for display. All trained model artifacts are serialized as Python pickle files with a standardized dictionary structure (model, scaler, features), enabling seamless loading, version tracking, and reproducibility (Table 5.15).

Figure 5.16 presents the LungAI-Dx Streamlit application dashboard across three views. The dashboard serves as the primary entry point to the platform, providing clinicians and researchers with an immediate overview of the dataset scope, computational pipeline architecture, available analytical modules, and a gallery of key analytical figures generated by the framework.

Figure 5.17 illustrates the Lung Subtype Prediction module, which implements the XGBoost three-class classifier for NSCLC molecular subtype discrimination. The module accepts gene expression input through three modes (manual entry, CSV upload, or random sample generation), produces calibrated class probability predictions, and provides patient-level SHAP explanations identifying the transcriptomic features most influential in each classification decision.

Table 5.15 LungAI-Dx Streamlit application module summary

Module	Page title	Primary function	Key outputs
1	Dashboard	Project overview, dataset summary, key metrics	Summary statistics, pipeline overview
2	Lung subtype prediction	XGBoost 3-class classification from expression CSV	Predicted subtype, class probabilities, SHAP explanation
3	Clinical risk assessment	Rule-based and logistic risk scoring	Recurrence risk score, mortality risk tier
4	Survival prediction	KM curves + Cox PI individual risk estimate	PI risk group (Low/Int/High), simulated survival curve
5	Biomarker profile	TMB calculator, mutation status, methylation	TMB tier, IO eligibility, methylation summary
6	Drug recommendations	DGIdb + IO eligibility matching engine	FDA-approved therapy list, clinical trial references
7	Model performance	All classifier metrics, ROC curves, SHAP	CV/test metric tables, AUC heatmap, confusion matrix
8	Batch analysis	Multi-sample bulk prediction and risk scoring	Batch prediction CSV, bulk risk score download
9	SaMD framework	Regulatory classification and risk management	IMDRF/FDA/EU MDR classification, IEC/ISO risk tables

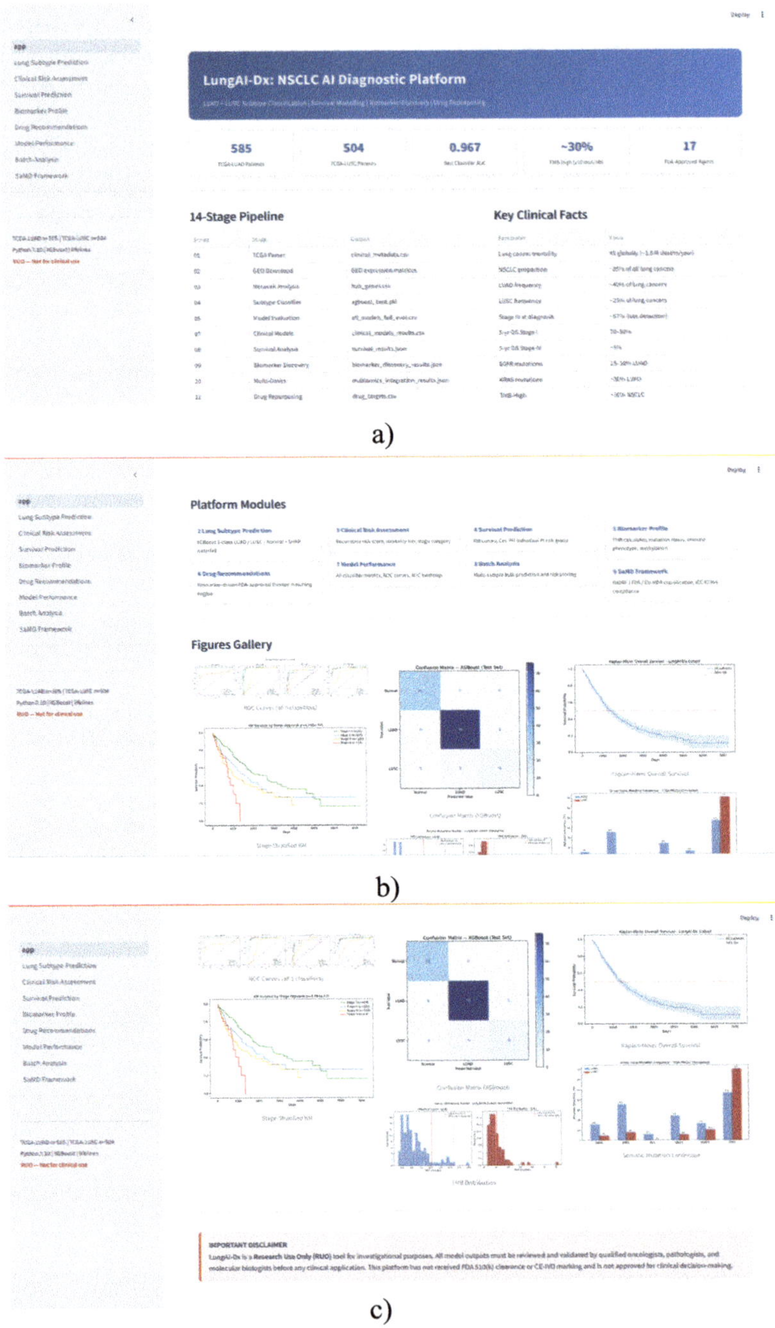

Fig. 5.16 LungAI-Dx Dashboard, **a** main landing page with platform summary statistics, 14-stage pipeline overview, and key clinical facts reference tab, **b** Platform Modules overview with nine interactive module cards and embedded Figures Gallery showing key analytical visualizations, **c** Figures Gallery continuation with key analytical visualizations and Research Use Only (RUO) disclaimer

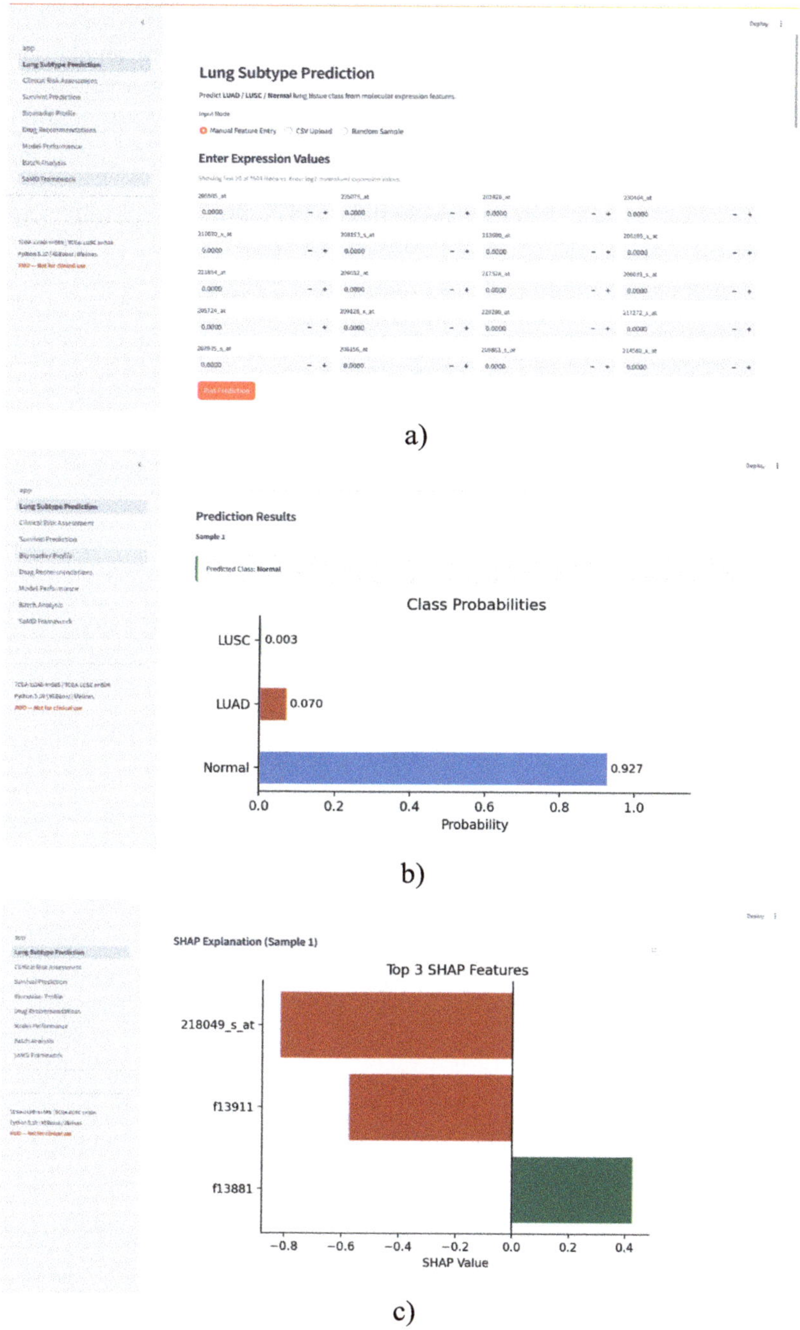

Fig. 5.17 Lung Subtype Prediction Module **a** manual feature entry input interface for 9904 Affymetrix probe expression values with three input modes (manual, CSV upload, random sample), **b** prediction results displaying predicted class (Normal) with calibrated class probability bar chart, **c** SHAP explanation showing the top 3 transcriptomic features driving the individual classification decision with directional SHAP values

Figure 5.18 demonstrates the clinical risk assessment module, which computes rule-based recurrence risk, five-year mortality risk, and stage classification from standard clinical parameters. The module provides an intuitive input interface for clinical variables and returns a comprehensive risk profile with overall risk tier stratification and evidence-based clinical recommendations.

Figure 5.19 presents the Survival Prediction module, which translates the Cox proportional hazards model and Prognostic Index (PI) framework into an interactive

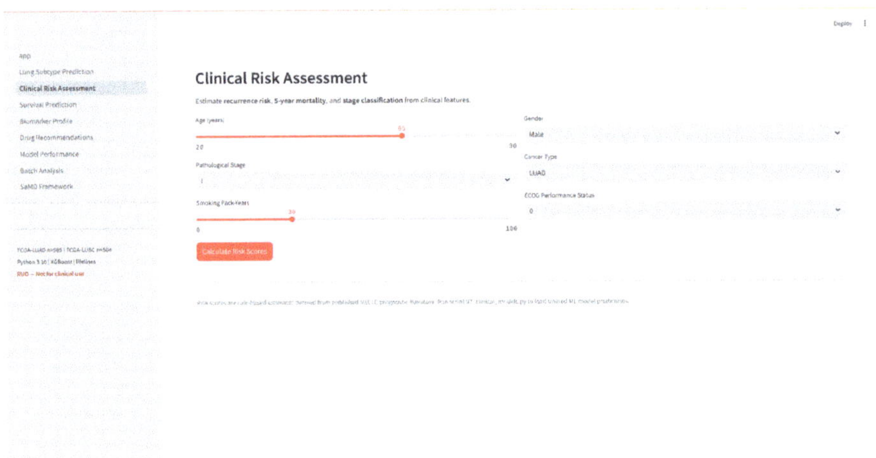

a)

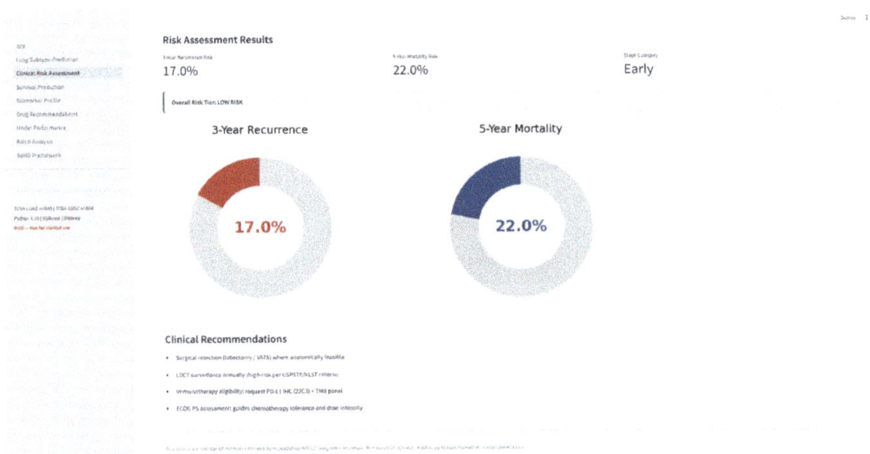

b)

Fig. 5.18 Clinical risk assessment module **a** clinical parameter input interface with age, pathological stage, smoking pack-years, gender, cancer type, and ECOG performance status controls, **b** results showing risk scores, stage category, overall risk tier (LOW RISK), donut chart visualizations, and evidence-based clinical recommendations

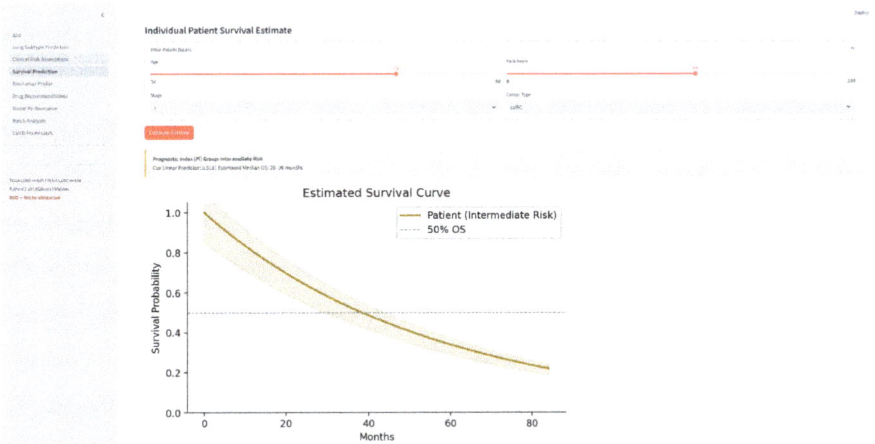

Fig. 5.19 Survival Prediction Module, individual patient survival estimate showing clinical input parameters, Prognostic Index (PI) group assignment (intermediate risk), Cox linear predictor value, estimated median OS, and personalized survival curve with confidence interval

patient-level survival estimation tool. Clinicians enter patient-specific clinical parameters and receive an individualized survival curve with confidence bands, PI risk group classification, and estimated median overall survival, enabling personalized prognostic counseling.

Figure 5.20 illustrates the drug recommendations module, which implements the pharmacogenomic decision-support engine. The module accepts a comprehensive patient biomarker profile including actionable mutations, TMB, PD-L1 expression, and treatment context and generates a prioritized list of FDA-approved targeted therapies and immunotherapy regimens with supporting clinical trial references and evidence levels.

5.6 Limitations and Future Directions

While LungAI-Dx demonstrates strong analytical performance and clinical relevance, several methodological and translational limitations must be acknowledged to contextualize its findings appropriately. This section first enumerates the key constraints of the current framework including dataset biases, class imbalance, temporal gaps, and regulatory status and then outlines the future research directions that would address these limitations and advance the platform toward prospective clinical deployment.

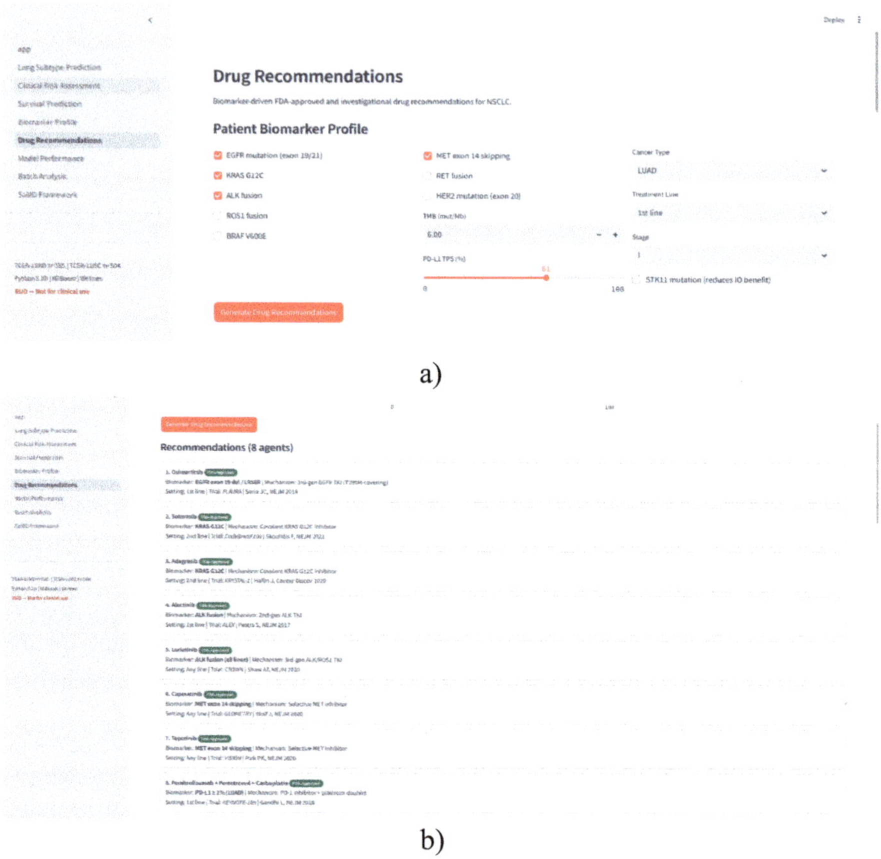

Fig. 5.20 Drug recommendations module **a** patient biomarker profile input interface with actionable mutation checkboxes, TMB, PD-L1 TPS, and treatment context parameters, **b** output displaying 8 prioritized FDA-approved agents with biomarker targets, mechanisms of action, treatment settings, and pivotal clinical trial references

5.6.1 Limitations

- **Training Data Bias**: GEO cohorts are enriched for early-stage, surgically resected tumors from North American and Japanese academic centers. Performance in community-practice settings with late-stage and biopsy-limited specimens requires prospective validation in demographically diverse cohorts.
- **LUSC Underrepresentation**: Only 43 LUSC samples (7.4%) in the expression dataset mean that the LUSC classifier is trained partially on synthetic BorderlineSMOTE-2 samples. LUSC-specific performance may be unreliable in independent cohorts with greater squamous cell histological diversity.

- **Temporal Validation Gap**: TCGA clinical data were collected 2009–2016, prior to widespread adoption of osimertinib (FDA 2015) and pembrolizumab (FDA 2016). Survival estimates may not reflect outcomes achievable with modern targeted and immunotherapy regimens.
- **Platform Harmonization**: The primary classifier accepts Affymetrix HG-U133Plus2 microarray profiles. RNA sequencing, the current clinical standard requires probe-to-gene-level harmonization steps before the trained model can be applied, which may introduce measurement platform bias.
- **Research Use Only Status**: LungAI-Dx has not undergone prospective clinical validation or regulatory review. All outputs are research use only and must not be used to inform clinical decisions without independent validation and regulatory approval.

5.6.2 Future Directions

Several methodologically distinct and clinically significant extensions are envisaged: (i) integration of pathology whole-slide image features through a multimodal classifier combining transcriptomic and histopathological embeddings from a Vision Transformer architecture; (ii) longitudinal circulating tumor DNA (ctDNA) monitoring module for real-time treatment response tracking from serial liquid biopsy data; (iii) federated learning architecture enabling model training across multiple hospital sites without centralizing patient data, addressing both regulatory privacy requirements and dataset demographic diversity; (iv) prospective clinical trial integration, using LungAI-Dx as a biomarker-based stratification tool within an immunotherapy or targeted therapy trial design; and (v) large language model (LLM) integration for automated synthesis of patient-level genomic reports and multidisciplinary team decision-support summaries consistent with international oncology reporting standards.

5.7 Summary

This chapter has presented LungAI-Dx, a comprehensive end-to-end artificial intelligence framework for non-small cell lung cancer molecular subtype classification, survival prediction, biomarker discovery, multi-omics integration, and pharmacogenomic decision support. The framework integrates 583 GEO transcriptomic samples with clinical and genomic data from 1089 TCGA patients into a coherent analytical pipeline spanning 14 computational scripts and a nine-module interactive decision-support application.

The XGBoost classifier achieved a test-set macro-AUC of 0.9674, accuracy of 96.58%, and perfect binary sensitivity (1.0) for malignant tissue detection. MOFA-style PCA multi-omics integration improved AUC to 0.9699. Kaplan–Meier and

Cox survival analysis confirmed pathological stage as the dominant independent prognosticator (HR = 1.329, $p < 0.001$), while PI risk stratification revealed a 21.8 percentage-point separation in 5-year OS between high- and low-risk groups (log-rank $p = 2 \times 10^{-6}$). Biomarker analysis identified KRAS (36.0%) and EGFR (15.8%) as dominant actionable drivers, with 21.5% of patients eligible for pembrolizumab under TMB-High criteria. Drug-gene interaction analysis yielded 30 FDA-approved pharmacogenomic recommendations.

LungAI-Dx demonstrates the feasibility and clinical value of integrating machine learning, survival analysis, multi-omics, and pharmacogenomics within a single coherent decision-support platform. The framework provides a validated, open, and extensible foundation for prospective clinical evaluation and future regulatory submission in precision oncology settings worldwide.

References

1. Sung, H., Ferlay, J., Siegel, R. L., Laversanne, M., Soerjomataram, I., Jemal, A., & Bray, F. (2021). Global cancer statistics 2020: GLOBOCAN estimates of incidence and mortality worldwide for 36 cancers in 185 countries. *CA: A Cancer Journal for Clinicians, 71*(3), 209–249.
2. Siegel, R. L., Miller, K. D., Wagle, N. S., & Jemal, A. (2023). Cancer statistics, 2023. *CA: A Cancer Journal for Clinicians, 73*(1), 17–48.
3. Howlader, N. N., Noone, A. M., Krapcho, M. E., Miller, D., Brest, A., Yu, M. E., Cronin, K., et al. (2019). SEER cancer statistics review, 1975–2016. *National Cancer Institute, 1.*
4. Subramanian, J., & Govindan, R. (2007). Lung cancer in never smokers: A review. *Journal of Clinical Oncology, 25*(5), 561–570.
5. Travis, W. D., Brambilla, E., Nicholson, A. G., Yatabe, Y., Austin, J. H., Beasley, M. B., Chirieac, L. R., Dacic, S., Duhig, E., Flieder, D. B., Geisinger, K., & Wistuba, I. (2015). The 2015 World Health Organization classification of lung tumors: Impact of genetic, clinical and radiologic advances since the 2004 classification. *Journal of Thoracic Oncology, 10*(9), 1243–1260.
6. Soria, J. C., Ohe, Y., Vansteenkiste, J., Reungwetwattana, T., Chewaskulyong, B., Lee, K. H., Dechaphunkul, A., Imamura, F., Nogami, N., Kurata, T., Okamoto, I., & Ramalingam, S. S. (2018). Osimertinib in untreated EGFR-mutated advanced non–small-cell lung cancer. *New England Journal of Medicine, 378*(2), 113–125.
7. Gandara, D. R., Hammerman, P. S., Sos, M. L., Lara, P. N., Jr., & Hirsch, F. R. (2015). Squamous cell lung cancer: From tumor genomics to cancer therapeutics. *Clinical Cancer Research, 21*(10), 2236–2243.
8. Kourou, K., Exarchos, T. P., Exarchos, K. P., Karamouzis, M. V., & Fotiadis, D. I. (2015). Machine learning applications in cancer prognosis and prediction. *Computational and Structural Biotechnology Journal, 13*, 8–17.
9. Chen, J. H., & Asch, S. M. (2017). Machine learning and prediction in medicine—Beyond the peak of inflated expectations. *The New England Journal of Medicine, 376*(26), 2507.
10. Bibault, J. E., Giraud, P., & Burgun, A. (2016). Big data and machine learning in radiation oncology: State of the art and future prospects. *Cancer Letters, 382*(1), 110–117.
11. Bhattacharjee, A., Richards, W. G., Staunton, J., Li, C., Monti, S., Vasa, P., Ladd, C., Beheshti, J., Bueno, R., Gillette, M., Loda, M., Meyerson, M., et al. (2001). Classification of human lung carcinomas by mRNA expression profiling reveals distinct adenocarcinoma subclasses. *Proceedings of the National Academy of Sciences, 98*(24), 13790–13795.

12. Johnson, W. E., Li, C., & Rabinovic, A. (2007). Adjusting batch effects in microarray expression data using empirical Bayes methods. *Biostatistics, 8*(1), 118–127.
13. Coudray, N., Ocampo, P. S., Sakellaropoulos, T., Narula, N., Snuderl, M., Fenyö, D., Moreira, A.L., Razavian, N., & Tsirigos, A. (2018). Classification and mutation prediction from non–small cell lung cancer histopathology images using deep learning. *Nature Medicine, 24*(10), 1559–1567.
14. Kaplan, E. L., & Meier, P. (1958). Nonparametric estimation from incomplete observations. *Journal of the American Statistical Association, 53*(282), 457–481.
15. Ishwaran, H., Kogalur, U. B., Blackstone, E. H., & Lauer, M. S. (2008). Random survival forests.
16. Wang, P., Li, Y., & Reddy, C. K. (2019). Machine learning for survival analysis: A survey. *ACM Computing Surveys (CSUR), 51*(6), 1–36.
17. Subramanian, I., Verma, S., Kumar, S., Jere, A., & Anamika, K. (2020). Multi-omics data integration, interpretation, and its application. *Bioinformatics and Biology Insights, 14*, 1177932219899051.
18. Huang, S., Chaudhary, K., & Garmire, L. X. (2017). More is better: Recent progress in multi-omics data integration methods. *Frontiers in Genetics, 8*, 84.
19. Argelaguet, R., Velten, B., Arnol, D., Dietrich, S., Zenz, T., Marioni, J. C., Buettner, F., Huber, W., & Stegle, O. (2018). Multi-omics factor analysis—A framework for unsupervised integration of multi-omics data sets. *Molecular Systems Biology, 14*(6), MSB178124.
20. Griffith, M., Griffith, O. L., Coffman, A. C., Weible, J. V., McMichael, J. F., Spies, N. C., Koval, J., Das, I., Callaway, M. B., Eldred, J. M., Miller, C. A., Wilson, R. K., et al. (2013). DGIdb: Mining the druggable genome. *Nature Methods, 10*(12), 1209–1210.
21. Lamb, J., Crawford, E. D., Peck, D., Modell, J. W., Blat, I. C., Wrobel, M. J., Lerner, J., Brunet, J. P., Subramanian, A., Ross, K. N., Reich, M., Golub, T. R., et al. (2006). The connectivity map: Using gene-expression signatures to connect small molecules, genes, and disease. *Science, 313*(5795), 1929–1935.
22. Samstein, R. M., Lee, C. H., Shoushtari, A. N., Hellmann, M. D., Shen, R., Janjigian, Y. Y., . Barron, D. A., Zehir, A., Jordan, E. J., Omuro, A., Kaley, T. J., Morris, L. G., et al. (2019). Tumor mutational load predicts survival after immunotherapy across multiple cancer types. *Nature Genetics, 51*(2), 202–206.
23. Chawla, N. V., Bowyer, K. W., Hall, L. O., & Kegelmeyer, W. P. (2002). SMOTE: Synthetic minority over-sampling technique. *Journal of Artificial Intelligence Research, 16*, 321–357.
24. Chen, T., & Guestrin, C. (2016, August). Xgboost: A scalable tree boosting system. In *Proceedings of the 22nd acm sigkdd international conference on knowledge discovery and data mining* (pp. 785–794).
25. Ke, G., Meng, Q., Finley, T., Wang, T., Chen, W., Ma, W., Ye, Q., & Liu, T. Y. (2017). Lightgbm: A highly efficient gradient boosting decision tree. *Advances in Neural Information Processing Systems, 30.*
26. Breiman, L. (2001). Random forests mach. *Learn, 45*(1), 5–32.
27. Cortes, C., & Vapnik, V. (1995). Support-vector networks. *Machine Learning, 20*(3), 273–297.
28. Akiba, T., Sano, S., Yanase, T., Ohta, T., & Koyama, M. (2019, July). Optuna: A next-generation hyperparameter optimization framework. In *Proceedings of the 25th ACM SIGKDD international conference on knowledge discovery & data mining* (pp. 2623–2631).
29. Davidson-Pilon, C. (2019). Lifelines: Survival analysis in Python. *Journal of Open Source Software, 4*(40), 1317.
30. Chen, R., Yang, L., Goodison, S., & Sun, Y. (2020). Deep-learning approach to identifying cancer subtypes using high-dimensional genomic data. *Bioinformatics, 36*(5), 1476–1483.
31. Ettinger, D. S., Wood, D. E., Aisner, D. L., Akerley, W., Bauman, J. R., Bharat, A., Bruno, D. S., Chang, J. Y., Chirieac, L. R., D'Amico, T. A. Dilling, T. J., Hughes, M., et al. (2021). NCCN guidelines insights: Non–small cell lung cancer, version 2.2021: Featured updates to the NCCN guidelines. *Journal of the National Comprehensive Cancer Network, 19*(3), 254–266.
32. Cancer Genome Atlas Research Network. (2014). Comprehensive molecular profiling of lung adenocarcinoma. *Nature, 511*(7511), 543.

33. Skoulidis, F., Goldberg, M. E., Greenawalt, D. M., Hellmann, M. D., Awad, M. M., Gainor, J. F., Schrock, A. B., Hartmaier, R. J., Trabucco, S. E., Gay, L., Ali, S. M., Elvin, J. A., Singal, G., Ross, J. S., Fabrizio, D., Szabo, P. M., Chang, H. Heymach, J. V., et al. (2018). STK11/LKB1 mutations and PD-1 inhibitor resistance in KRAS-mutant lung adenocarcinoma. *Cancer Discovery*, *8*(7), 822–835.
34. Hellmann, M. D., Ciuleanu, T. E., Pluzanski, A., Lee, J. S., Otterson, G. A., Audigier-Valette, C., Minenza, E., Linardou, H., Burgers, S., Salman, P., Borghaei, H., Ramalingam, S. S., Brahmer, J., Reck, M., O'Byrne, K. J., Geese, W. J., Green, G., Chang H., Paz-Ares, L., et al. (2018). Nivolumab plus ipilimumab in lung cancer with a high tumor mutational burden. *New England Journal of Medicine*, *378*(22), 2093–2104.
35. Binnewies, M., Roberts, E. W., Kersten, K., Chan, V., Fearon, D. F., Merad, M., Coussens, L. M., Gabrilovich, D. I., Ostrand-Rosenberg, S., Hedrick, C. C., Vonderheide, R. H., Krummel, M. F., et al. (2018). Understanding the tumor immune microenvironment (TIME) for effective therapy. *Nature Medicine*, *24*(5), 541–550.
36. Shia, J. (2008). Immunohistochemistry versus microsatellite instability testing for screening colorectal cancer patients at risk for hereditary nonpolyposis colorectal cancer syndrome: Part I. The utility of immunohistochemistry. *The Journal of Molecular Diagnostics*, *10*(4), 293–300.
37. Camidge, D. R., Kim, H. R., Ahn, M. J., Yang, J. C., Han, J. Y., Hochmair, M. J., Lee, K. H., Delmonte, A., Campelo, M. R. G., Kim, D. W., Griesinger, F., Felip, E., Califano, R., Spira, A. I., Gettinger, S, N., Tiseo, M., Lin, H. M., Liu, Y., Popat, S., et al. (2021). Brigatinib versus crizotinib in ALK inhibitor–naive advanced ALK-positive NSCLC: Final results of phase 3 ALTA-1L trial. *Journal of Thoracic Oncology*, *16*(12), 2091–2108.
38. Selamat, S. A., Chung, B. S., Girard, L., Zhang, W., Zhang, Y., Campan, M., Siegmund, K. D., Koss, M. N., Hagen, J. A., Lam, W. L., Lam, S., Gazdar, A, F., & Laird-Offringa, I. A. (2012). Genome-scale analysis of DNA methylation in lung adenocarcinoma and integration with mRNA expression. *Genome Research*, *22*(7), 1197–1211.

Chapter 6
The Lung Cancer Risk Prediction (LCRP) Agent

This chapter presents a detailed case study of the Lung Cancer Risk Prediction (LCRP) Agent, a Streamlit-based, machine-learning-powered clinical decision-support tool that provides preliminary lung cancer risk assessments from patient-reported health and lifestyle data. The LCRP Agent is the foundational module of the multi-agent lung cancer AI ecosystem developed in this book. It operates exclusively on structured clinical tabular data, requiring no imaging, and serves as the first-pass risk-screening layer in the broader diagnostic pipeline.

6.1 Introduction and Clinical Motivation

Lung cancer is the leading cause of cancer-related mortality worldwide, responsible for approximately 1.8 million deaths annually [1]. Survival rates exceed 60% for stage I disease but fall below 10% for metastatic presentations, underscoring the critical importance of early detection [2]. The LCRP Agent was developed to address the gap in accessible, data-driven preliminary risk assessment, enabling clinicians and patients to identify high-risk individuals who warrant further radiological or pathological investigation, without requiring immediate access to imaging equipment or specialist facilities. The agent utilizes 16 clinical and lifestyle features, including smoking status, environmental exposures, respiratory symptoms, and family history to compute a personalized lung cancer risk probability through a trained Random Forest classifier. The output is a color-coded risk category and a downloadable structured HTML report, making it suitable for integration into primary care and telemedicine settings.

S. Shah and R. Thanki, *Artificial Intelligence for Early Detection and Diagnosis of Lung Cancer*, Signals and Communication Technology,
https://doi.org/10.1007/978-3-032-29615-3_6

6.2 System Architecture

The LCRP Agent is built on a two-tier architecture: a Streamlit web frontend and a Python ML backend. The backend loads a pre-trained RandomForestClassifier and a StandardScaler (both serialized as.joblib files) at application start. Patient data entered via the UI is numerically encoded, scaled, and passed to the model, which returns a probability score. The score is classified into one of four risk tiers, and a downloadable HTML report is generated. Case IDs are not auto generated in this agent, the user supplies Patient Name and ID directly.

6.3 Patient Input Features

The LCRP Agent collects 16 patient features covering demographics, lifestyle risk factors, symptom burden, and family history. Table 6.1 documents all feature with their input widget type and clinical rationale.

6.4 Model Development and Comparative Evaluation

Prior to deployment, three ensemble classifiers, Random Forest, Gradient Boosting, and XGBoost were evaluated in an MLOps pipeline on a held-out test set of 1000 patient records (593 Class 0: no cancer; 407 Class 1: cancer present). The Random Forest was selected as the deployment model based on its superior weighted F1-Score (0.9038) and overall accuracy (90.40%) [3]. Table 6.2 presents comparative evaluation for all three models. Table 6.3 provides per-class details for each model while Table 6.4 provides the risk category classification to make clinical action relevance.

6.5 User Interface of LCRP Agent

6.5.1 Patient Data Entry Interface

Figure 6.1a shows the upper portion of the LCRP Agent patient input form. The two-column layout presents sliders for continuous variables (Age: default 50; Oxygen Saturation: default 95%) and dropdown menus for binary and categorical variables (Gender: Male; Smoking Status: Non-Smoker; all binary risk factors defaulting to No). This approach minimizes free-text entry and enforces data consistency. Figure 6.2b shows the lower portion of the input form, revealing the remaining fields, History of Long-Term Illness, Family History of Lung Cancer, Energy Level

Table 6.1 Patient input features collected by the LCRP agent

Feature	Input widget/Range	Clinical rationale
Age	Slider 18–100	Biological age—strongest independent risk predictor
Gender	Dropdown: Male/Female	Sex-based epidemiological risk stratification
Smoking status	Dropdown: Non-Smoker/ Smoker/Former	Primary modifiable lung cancer risk factor
Finger discoloration	Dropdown: Yes/No	Peripheral nicotine staining – heavy smoking indicator
Mental stress	Dropdown: Yes/No	Psychosocial risk factor associated with immune suppression
Exposure to pollution	Dropdown: Yes / No	Occupational / environmental carcinogen exposure
History of long-term illness	Dropdown: Yes/No	Chronic comorbidity flag (COPD, fibrosis)
Energy level (%)	Slider 0–100	Self-reported vitality—fatigue as a symptom proxy
Immune system weakness	Dropdown: Yes/No	Immunocompromised status
Breathing issues	Dropdown: Yes/No	Dyspnea or recurrent respiratory symptoms
Consumes alcohol	Dropdown: Yes/No	Alcohol-lung cancer risk co-factor
Throat discomfort	Dropdown: Yes/No	Persistent hoarseness or irritation
Oxygen saturation (%)	Slider 90–100	Resting peripheral SpO_2
Chest tightness or pain	Dropdown: Yes/No	Thoracic symptom flag
Family history of lung cancer	Dropdown: Yes/No	First-degree genetic risk factor
Family members who smoke	Dropdown: Yes/No	Passive smoke/second-hand exposure

Table 6.2 MLOps model comparison: random forest, gradient boosting, XGBoost

Model	Accuracy	Precision (Wt.)	F1-score (Wt.)	ROC AUC
Random forest	0.9040	0.9038	0.9038	0.9232
Gradient boosting	0.8990	0.8989	0.8989	0.9237
XGBoost	0.8850	0.8849	0.8849	0.9095

Table 6.3 Per-class classification report for all three models (test set)

Model	Class	Precision	Recall	F1-Score
Random forest	Class 0 (no cancer)	0.9135	0.9258	0.9196
Random forest	Class 1 (cancer)	0.8897	0.8722	0.8809
Gradient boosting	Class 0 (no cancer)	0.9114	0.9191	0.9152
Gradient boosting	Class 1 (cancer)	0.8806	0.8698	0.8752
XGBoost	Class 0 (no cancer)	0.8997	0.9073	0.9034
XGBoost	Class 1 (cancer)	0.8632	0.8526	0.8578

Table 6.4 Risk category classification scheme

Category	Range (%)	Color	Clinical action
Low	0–25	Green	Low statistical probability; standard preventive follow-up
Medium	26–50	Amber	Moderate risk; additional clinical evaluation recommended
High	51–75	Orange	Elevated risk; specialist referral and imaging workup warranted
Critical	76–100	Red	Very high risk; immediate specialist consultation required

slide (default 50%), and Family Members Who Smoke. The ‘Analyze Patient Data’ button and the educational-use disclaimer are visible at the bottom of the form.

6.5.2 *Post-Prediction Interface and Risk Assessment Result Display*

Figure 6.2a shows the complete input form preserved in the post-prediction state, confirming all entered values remain visible for clinician review and auditability. Inputs reflect the illustrative default profile: Age 50, Male, Non-Smoker, all binary risk factors No, Oxygen Saturation 95%, Energy Level 50%. Figure 6.2b shows the Risk Assessment Result panel. For the illustrative default profile, the agent returned: Risk Category: Low, Predicted Risk Percentage: 6.00%, Interpretation: Low risk of lung cancer. A ‘Download Full Report (.html)’ button is provided for record integration.

6.6 Generated Report

Figure 6.3 presents the generated Lung Cancer Risk Prediction Report (HTML) for the illustrative case (Case ID: LUNG20250813161529). The report contains two sections: (1) Patient Input Features: a tabular listing of all 16 entered values; (2)

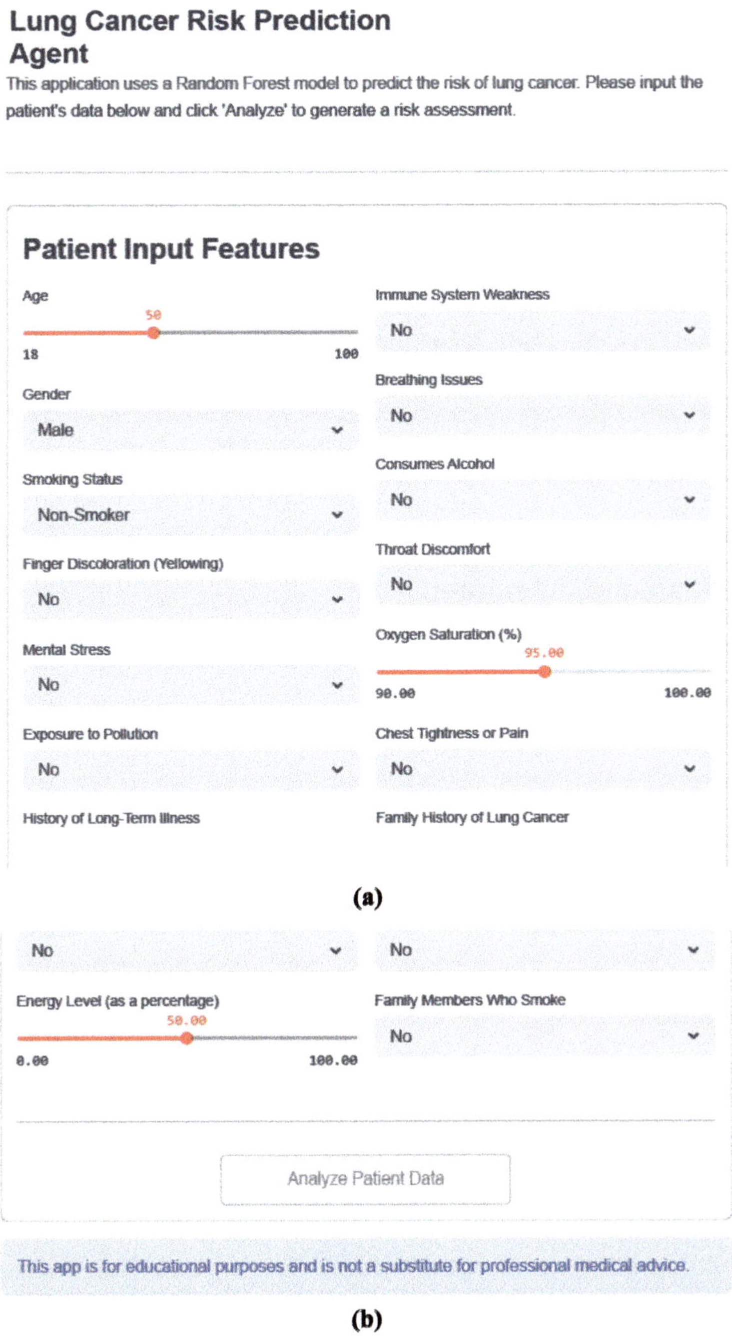

Fig. 6.1 LCRP agent patient data entry interface **a** upper section of the LCRP agent patient input form. Demographic and primary symptom fields with slider and dropdown widgets **b** lower section of the LCRP Agent patient input form, with remaining risk factor fields, 'Analyze Patient Data' button, and educational disclaimer

Prediction Result: Risk Category: Low; Predicted Risk Percentage: 6.00%; Interpretation: Low risk of lung cancer. A centered disclaimer clarifies the report is AI-generated for informational purposes only.

- **Key observations of illustrative case (anonymous, LUNG20250813161529)**
  - **Profile**: Male, Age 50, non-smoker; no binary risk factors present; SpO_2 95%; energy level 50%.
  - **Result**: Risk category = low; predicted risk percentage = 6.00%.

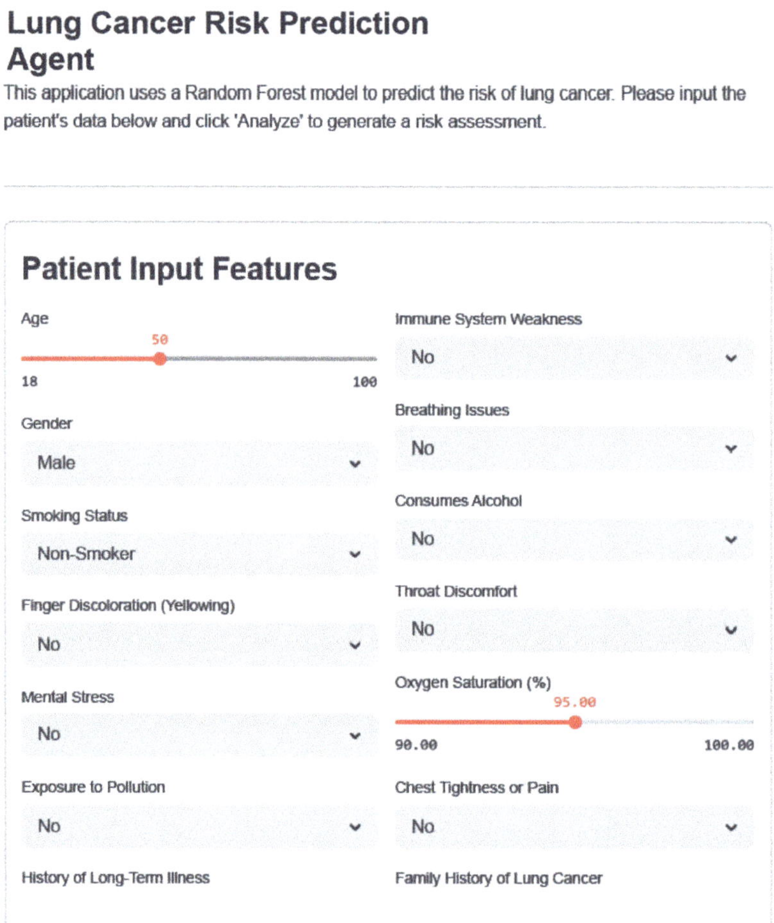

(a)

Fig. 6.2 LCRP agent post-prediction interface and risk assessment result **a** LCRP agent input form in post-prediction state. All entered values preserved for audit. Default profile: Age 50, Male, non-smoker, SpO_2 95%, energy level 50%. **b** LCRP agent risk assessment result: Risk category = low, predicted risk = 6.00%. Download full report button visible

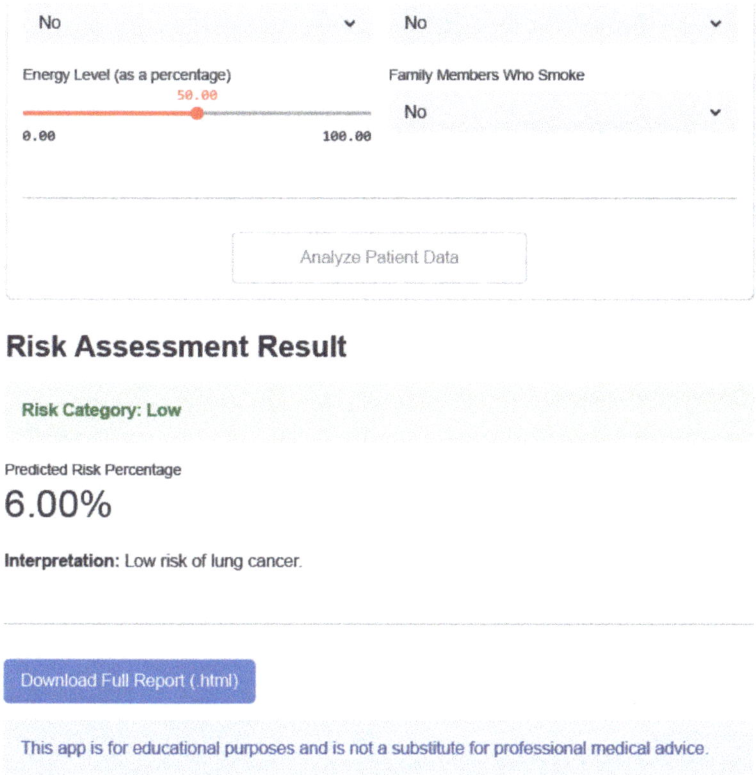

(b)

Fig. 6.2 (continued)

- **Clinical Logic**: Absence of smoking, respiratory symptoms, family history, and pollution exposure drives low prediction.
- **Output**: Downloadable HTML report generated for EHR integration.
- **Disclaimer**: For educational purposes; not a substitute for clinical diagnosis.

6.7 Summary

The LCRP Agent establishes the foundational risk-screening layer of the multi-agent AI diagnostic ecosystem. Its Random Forest model (accuracy: 90.40%, F1: 0.9038) provides a reliable first-pass assessment from structured clinical data alone, making it deployable in settings without imaging infrastructure [4]. Limitations include reliance on self-reported data (susceptible to recall bias) and the moderate validation accuracy that is inherent to tabular clinical data classification. Future enhancements

Lung Cancer Risk Prediction Report

Date: 2025-08-13 16:15:29

Patient Input Features

Feature	Value
Age	50
Gender	Male
Smoking Status	Non-Smoker
Finger Discoloration (Yellowing)	No
Mental Stress	No
Exposure to Pollution	No
History of Long-Term Illness	No
Energy Level (as a percentage)	50.00
Immune System Weakness	No
Breathing Issues	No
Consumes Alcohol	No
Throat Discomfort	No
Oxygen Saturation (%)	95.00
Chest Tightness or Pain	No
Family History of Lung Cancer	No
Family Members Who Smoke	No

Prediction Result

Risk Category: Low

Predicted Risk Percentage: 6.00%

Interpretation: Low risk of lung cancer.

Disclaimer: This report is generated by an AI agent and is for informational purposes only. It is not a substitute for professional medical advice, diagnosis, or treatment.

Fig. 6.3 Generated LCRP agent lung cancer risk prediction report

include integration of genomic risk scores, FHIR-compatible EHR data ingestion, and uncertainty quantification through conformal prediction [5]. The LCRP Agent serves as the clinical risk quantification input to the multimodal MLCA Agent (Chap. 8), where its risk score is synthesized alongside CT and histopathology findings by a Generative AI model to produce a holistic diagnostic report.

References

1. WHO. (2023). *Global cancer observatory: Cancer today*. IARC.
2. Siegel, R. L., Miller, K. D., Wagle, N. S., & Jemal, A. (2023). Cancer statistics, 2023. *CA: A Cancer Journal for Clinicians, 73*(1), 17–48.
3. Parikh, R. B., Teeple, S., & Navathe, A. S. (2019). Addressing bias in artificial intelligence in health care. *JAMA, 322*(24), 2377–2378.
4. Topol, E. J. (2019). High-performance medicine: The convergence of human and artificial intelligence. *Nature Medicine, 25*(1), 44–56.
5. Kompa, B., Snoek, J., & Beam, A. L. (2021). Second opinion needed: Communicating uncertainty in medical machine learning. *NPJ Digital Medicine, 4*(1), 4.

Chapter 7
CT and Histopathology Imaging AI Agents: HieraLung and HistoLung

This chapter presents two AI diagnostic agents that analyze lung cancer imaging data at different modalities and stages of the clinical pathway: the HieraLung Diagnostic Agent (Sects. 7.1–7.6), which performs hierarchical CT scan classification, and the HistoLung Diagnostic Agent (Sects. 7.7–7.11), which classifies lung histopathology H&E slides. Together, these two agents provide radiological and pathological AI-assisted decision support, forming the imaging intelligence core of the multi-agent lung cancer diagnostic ecosystem.

Part A: The HieraLung Diagnostic Agent

7.1 Introduction to HieraLung

The HieraLung Diagnostic Agent addresses the radiological analysis stage of lung cancer diagnosis through a two-stage hierarchical inference pipeline applied to CT scan images. Stage 1 (triage) classifies CT images as Normal, Benign, or Malignant using a CNN triage model. Only images classified as Malignant proceed to Stage 2 (Subtype), where a second CNN identifies the specific cancer subtype (adenocarcinoma, large cell carcinoma, or squamous cell carcinoma). This hierarchical approach mirrors the clinical pathway from radiological triage to pathological sub-classification [1], improving computational efficiency by invoking the more specialized subtype model only when clinically warranted.

S. Shah and R. Thanki, *Artificial Intelligence for Early Detection and Diagnosis of Lung Cancer*, Signals and Communication Technology,
https://doi.org/10.1007/978-3-032-29615-3_7

7.2 System Architecture and Pipeline

The HieraLung Agent is deployed as a Streamlit web application with a split-panel interface. The left sidebar collects Case Information (Patient Name, auto-generated Case ID) and hosts the CT scan file uploader. Upon clicking "Run Diagnosis," the agent preprocesses the CT image to 224 × 224 pixels, passes it through the LC_Cases_Classifier (VGG16-based triage), and if Malignant then subsequently through the CNN LC_Types_Classifier (subtype). Results are displayed in the Diagnostic Summary panel, and a structured HTML report is offered for download.

7.2.1 Application Flowchart

Figure 7.1 shows the HieraLung application flowchart. Following image upload, the CT image is preprocessed and passed to the Stage 1 triage model. A Normal or Benign result concludes with the pipeline; a Malignant result activates the Stage 2 subtype model. All pathways converge at report generation and display.

7.2.2 Data Flow Diagram

Figure 7.2 presents the 12-step sequence data flow diagram showing how data move between User, UI, Agent, and Models components. Steps 1–5 cover CT upload and triage prediction; Steps 6–8 cover conditional subtype prediction; Steps 9–12 cover report compilation and delivery to the clinician.

7.3 Dataset Used for Development of HieraLung Agent

The HieraLung Agent is trained on the IQ-OTH/NCCD Lung Cancer Dataset [2], a publicly available CT scan dataset collected at the Iraq-Oncology Teaching Hospital and the National Center for Cancer Diseases (Baghdad, Iraq) during autumn 2019. The dataset contains 1,190 CT scan slice images derived from 110 clinical cases, categorized into three classes: Normal (55 cases, 416 images), Benign (15 cases, 120 images), and Malignant (40 cases, 561 images). All images were originally acquired in DICOM format using a Siemens SOMATOM scanner with a 120 kV tube voltage and 1 mm slice thickness, with window width ranging from 350 to 1200 HU and window center from 50 to 600 HU. The scans were annotated and validated by board-certified oncologists and radiologists at both institutions. The HieraLung Agent employs two distinct CT scan datasets (as given in Table 7.1 and Table 7.2) for its two-stage hierarchical pipeline, each class-balanced through augmentation to

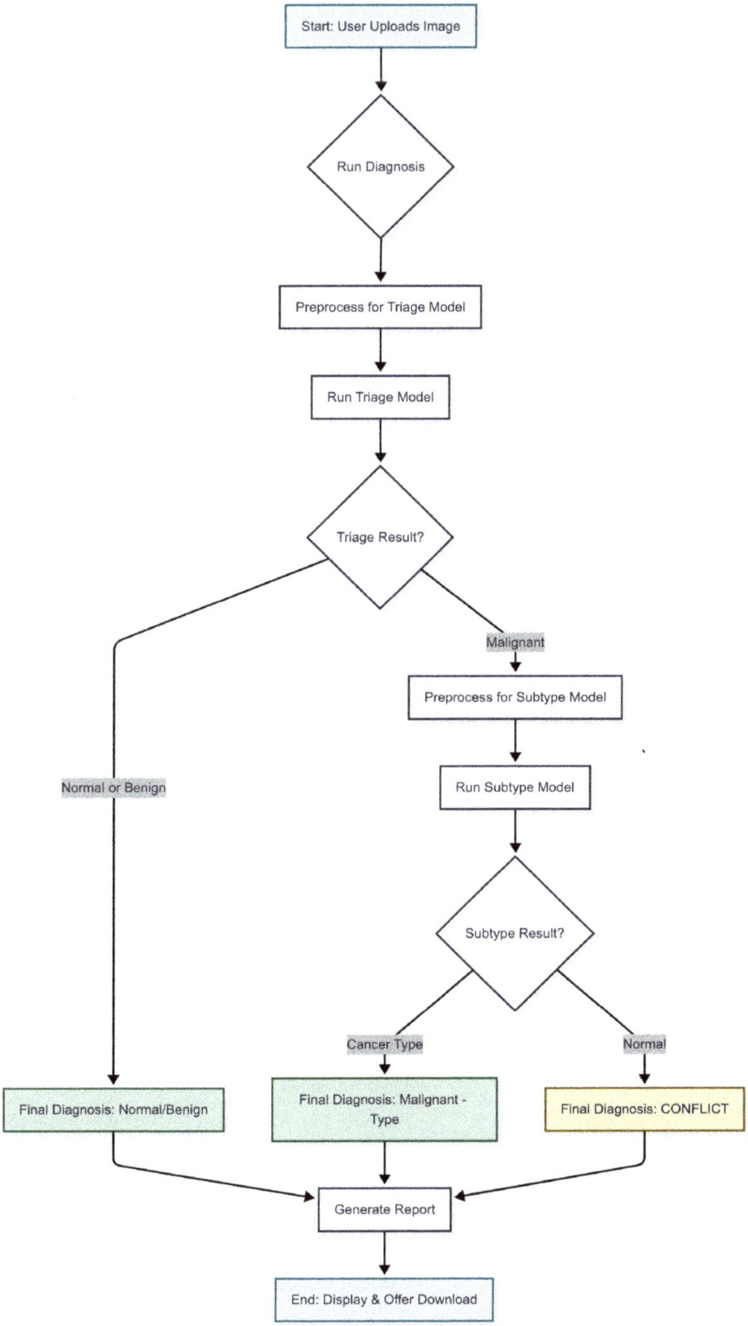

Fig. 7.1 HieraLung application flowchart: two-stage hierarchical diagnostic logic gating subtype classification on malignancy detection

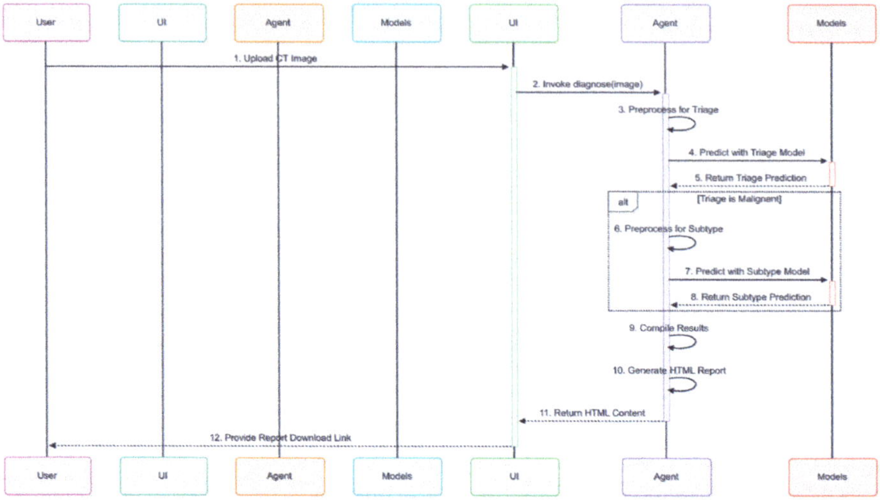

Fig. 7.2 HieraLung 12-step data flow sequence diagram (User → UI → Agent → Models)

ensure equitable training representation across all diagnostic categories. Table 7.1 shows the balance of dataset summary used for HieraLung triage model (LC_Cases_Classifier) training and validation.

For the Stage 2 subtype classification, the HieraLung Agent uses a separate balanced version of the Chest CT-scan dataset generated from the original

Table 7.1 Balanced IQ-OTH/NCCD dataset summary for HieraLung triage model (LC_Cases_Classifier) training and validation

Attribute	Details
Source and collection period	Iraq-Oncology Teaching Hospital/National Center for Cancer Diseases, Baghdad, Iraq, and Autumn 2019
Modality	Chest CT scan (DICOM, Siemens SOMATOM, 120 kV, 1 mm slice thickness)
Original total images	1190 images/110 cases (PNG format)
Original class distribution	Benign (15), Malignant (40), and Normal (55)
Balancing method	Augmentation (rotation, flipping, brightness adjustment) to equalize class counts
Class distribution after balancing method	Benign (10,000), Malignant (10,000), and Normal (10,000)
Preprocessing	Resized to 224 × 224 px; pixel values normalized to [0, 1]
Split strategy	80% training/20% validation
Annotation	Board-certified oncologists and radiologists

Table 7.2 Balanced chest CT scan images dataset summary for HieraLung subtype model (LC_Types_Classifier) training and validation

Attribute	Details
Dataset name	Balanced chest CT scan images dataset (lung CT scan dataset)
Modality	Chest CT scan images (PNG format)
Original total images	1000 CT images (pre-balanced)
Original class distribution	Adenocarcinoma (338), large cell carcinoma (187), squamous cell carcinoma (260), normal (215)
Balancing method	Augmentation (rotation, flipping, brightness adjustment) to equalize class counts
Class distribution after balancing method	Adenocarcinoma (10,000), large cell carcinoma (10,000), squamous cell carcinoma (10,000), normal (10,000)
Preprocessing	Resized to 224 × 224 px; pixel values normalized to [0, 1]
Split strategy	80% training/20% validation
Availability	www.kaggle.com/datasets/mohamedhanyyy/chest-ctscan-images (public) [3]

IQ-OTH/NCCD dataset [3], which compiled by Mohamed Hany, as summarized in Table 7.2. The original dataset contains 1,000 CT scan images across four classes: adenocarcinoma (338 images), large cell carcinoma (187 images), squamous cell carcinoma (260 images), and normal (215 images). To address the significant class imbalance, augmentation techniques (rotation, flipping, brightness adjustment) were applied to equalize class representation, producing the Balanced Lung CT Scan Dataset used for training. Images were resized to 224 × 224 pixels and normalized to [0, 1] for model input.

7.4 CNN Model Architecture and Performance

Tables 7.3 and 7.4 shows the lays out the convolutional neural network used by Triage model and Subtype model of HieraLung. It's a straightforward sequential CNN: three convolutional layers (32 → 64 → 128 filters) each followed by max-pooling to progressively extract and downsample spatial features from 224 × 224 CT images, then a flatten layer converts the 3D feature maps into a 1D vector of 100,352 features, which feeds into a 512-unit dense layer (where the bulk of the ~ 51 M parameters live), a dropout layer for regularization, and finally a task-specific output head 3 neurons for triage (Benign/Malignant/Normal) or 4 neurons for subtype (ACA/LCC/Normal/SCC). The key design choice is that both models share the same feature extraction backbone, differing only at the final classification layer.

Table 7.3 CNN architecture used by HieraLung triage model, total trainable parameters: 51,475,523

Layer	Output shape	Parameters	Function
conv2d (Conv2D)	(None, 224, 224, 32)	896	Feature extraction from raw CT image
max_pooling2d	(None, 112, 112, 32)	0	Spatial downsampling (2 × 2)
conv2d_1	(None, 112, 112, 64)	18,496	Intermediate feature map
max_pooling2d_1	(None, 56, 56, 64)	0	Spatial downsampling (2 × 2)
conv2d_2	(None, 56, 56, 128)	73,856	High-level feature extraction
max_pooling2d_2	(None, 28, 28, 128)	0	Final downsampling
flatten	(None, 100,352)	0	3D → 1D feature vector
dense (Dense)	(None, 512)	51,380,736	Fully connected classification head
dropout	(None, 512)	0	Regularization
dense_1 (Triage)	(None, 3)	1,539	Output: Benign / Malignant / Normal

Table 7.4 CNN architecture used by HieraLung subtype model, total trainable parameters: 51,476,036

Layer	Output shape	Parameters	Function
conv2d (Conv2D)	(None, 224, 224, 32)	896	Feature extraction from raw CT image
max_pooling2d	(None, 112, 112, 32)	0	Spatial downsampling (2 × 2)
conv2d_1	(None, 112, 112, 64)	18,496	Intermediate feature map
max_pooling2d_1	(None, 56, 56, 64)	0	Spatial downsampling (2 × 2)
conv2d_2	(None, 56, 56, 128)	73,856	High-level feature extraction
max_pooling2d_2	(None, 28, 28, 128)	0	Final downsampling
flatten	(None, 100,352)	0	3D → 1D feature vector
dense (Dense)	(None, 512)	51,380,736	Fully connected classification head
dropout	(None, 512)	0	Regularization
dense_1 (Subtype)	(None, 4)	2,052	Output: ACA / LCC / Normal / SCC

Table 7.5 presents per-class precision, recall, and F1-score for both classifiers on their validation sets. The Triage model achieves a macro-average F1 of ~ 0.79 (78.82% accuracy), with Malignant showing high precision (0.95) but lower recall (0.73) meaning that it's confident when it flags malignancy but misses some cases while Normal class is the weakest performer. The Subtype model is considerably stronger at ~ 0.92 macro-average F1 (91.94% accuracy), with large cell carcinoma and Normal classes both exceeding 0.94 F1, and adenocarcinoma being the relatively hardest class to classify. This performance gap makes clinical sense: the Triage task (distinguishing benign vs. malignant vs. normal) is inherently harder than subtyping once malignancy is already established.

Table 7.6 defines the complete decision matrix of the hierarchical pipeline, how the Triage and Subtype model outputs combine into a final clinical diagnosis label.

Table 7.5 Validation-set classification reports for LC cases classifier

Model	Class	Precision	Recall	F1	Dataset
Triage (LC cases)	Benign	0.8225	0.8155	0.8190	Validation
Triage (LC cases)	Malignant	0.9493	0.7300	0.8253	Validation
Triage (LC cases)	Normal	0.6608	0.8190	0.7314	Validation
Triage (LC cases)	Macro avg	0.8108	0.7882	0.7919	Validation
Subtype (LC types)	Adenocarcinoma	0.8630	0.8440	0.8534	Validation
Subtype (LC types)	Large cell carc	0.9478	0.9350	0.9414	Validation
Subtype (LC types)	Normal	0.9777	0.9850	0.9813	Validation
Subtype (LC types)	Squamous cell carc	0.8886	0.9135	0.9009	Validation
Subtype (LC types)	Macro avg	0.9193	0.9194	0.9192	Validation

Normal and Benign triage results both map to a green-coded "Normal/Benign" output with routine follow-up. Malignant triage results cascade to the Subtype model, yielding red-coded outputs for adenocarcinoma (oncology referral), large cell carcinoma (urgent workup), or squamous cell carcinoma (bronchoscopy). The clever addition is the amber "CONFLICT" flag: if Triage says Malignant but Subtype says Normal (a logically inconsistent pair), the system defaults to Malignant as a safety measure and flags the case for human review, a patient-safety-first design decision that avoids false negatives at the cost of occasional over-referral.

7.5 User Interface of HieraLung Agent

7.5.1 Landing Screen

Figure 7.3 shows the HieraLung landing screen. The sidebar provides Case Information (Patient Name: Anonymous; auto-generated Case ID) and a CT scan file uploader. The main panel shows the title and an upload prompt.

Table 7.6 HieraLung diagnostic output categories and clinical action guidance

Triage × subtype result	Final diagnosis label	Color	Clinical action
Normal	Normal/Benign	Green	No malignant features; standard follow-up
Benign	Normal/Benign	Green	Benign nodule; clinical monitoring advised
Malignant → adenocarcinoma	Malignant (ACA)	Red	Most common NSCLC; oncology referral
Malignant → large cell carc	Malignant (LCC)	Red	Aggressive NSCLC; urgent workup required
Malignant → squamous cell carc	Malignant (SCC)	Red	Central airway NSCLC; bronchoscopy needed
Conflict (Triage = mal., Sub = Normal)	CONFLICT (Flag)	Amber	Defaults to Malignant; flags for human review

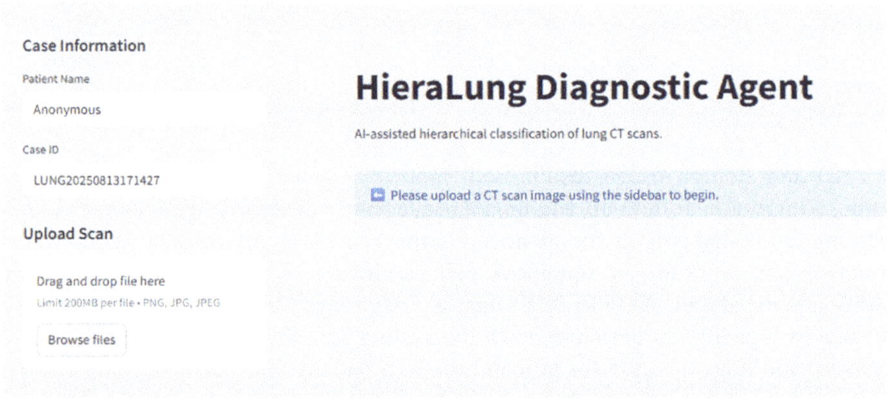

Fig. 7.3 HieraLung landing screen

7.5.2 Post-upload State

Figure 7.4 shows the interface after uploading lung CT image. The axial thoracic CT image is displayed in the left column. A “Run Diagnosis” button appears below the scan.

7.5.3 Post-prediction Results

Figure 7.5 shows the diagnostic summary after pipeline completion. Stage 1 Triage: malignant (100.0% confidence). Stage 2 Subtype: large cell carcinoma (100.0% confidence). Both scores are shown in green with upward arrows. “Download Full Report (HTML)” button is available.

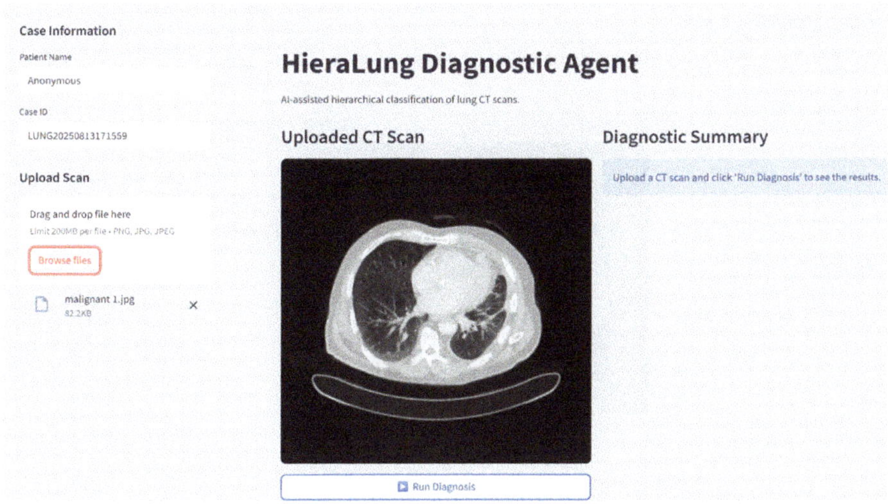

Fig. 7.4 HieraLung post-CT upload state

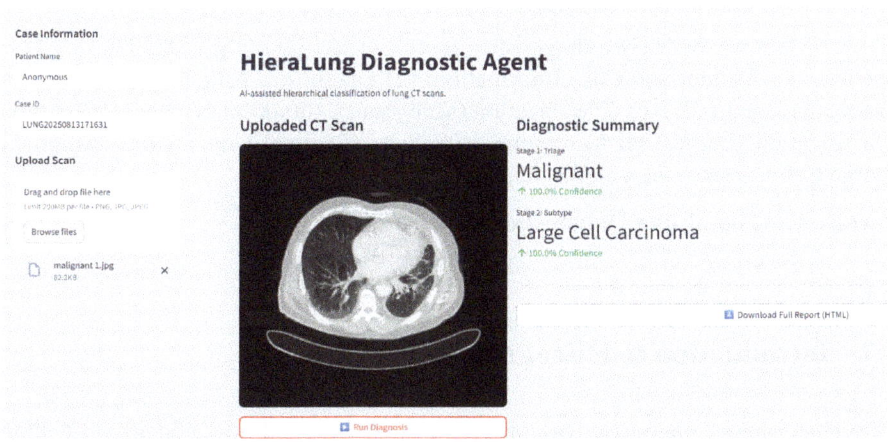

Fig. 7.5 HieraLung post-diagnosis results

7.5.4 Report Download State

Figure 7.6 captures the browser download notification (top right) confirming the HTML report download (HieraLung_Report_LUNG20250813171713.html).

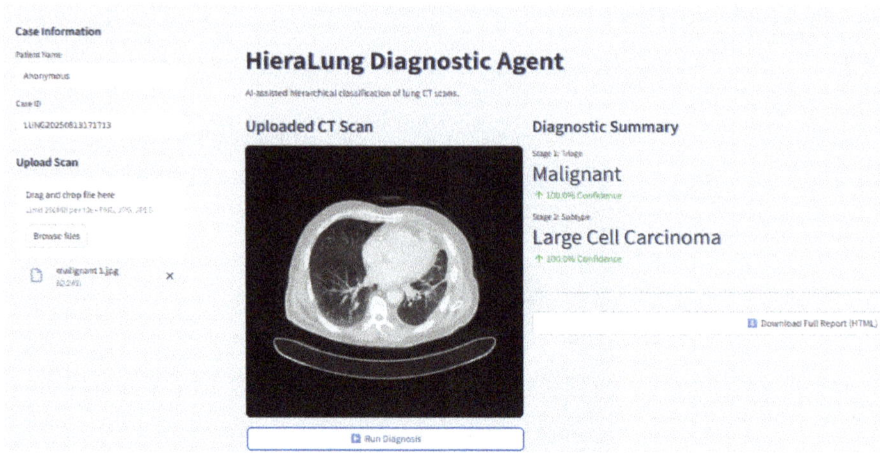

Fig. 7.6 HieraLung report download state

7.6 Generated HieraLung Report

Figure 7.7 shows the HTML diagnostic report for Case ID LUNG20250813172124. Sections: (1) Patient and Case Information; (2) Diagnostic Analysis with CT scan image; (3) Stage 1: Triage Classification (Malignant), 100.00%; (4) Stage 2: Subtype Classification (Large Cell Carcinoma), 99.96%; (5) Final Conclusion: Malignant (Large Cell Carcinoma); (6) Disclaimer.

Part B: The HistoLung Diagnostic Agent

7.7 Introduction to HistoLung

The HistoLung Diagnostic Agent provides AI-assisted classification of lung histopathology H&E-stained slide images. Histopathological examination of biopsy tissue remains the gold standard for lung cancer diagnosis [4]. The HistoLung Agent uses a single end-to-end CNN model to classify slides into three categories: lung adenocarcinoma (ACA), Lung Benign Tissue (BNT), and lung squamous cell carcinoma (SCC). Unlike the HieraLung Agent, the HistoLung pipeline is linear (no hierarchical branching), reflecting the direct classification nature of histopathology analysis from a single tissue specimen.

HieraLung Diagnostic Report

AI-Assisted Clinical Decision Support

Patient & Case Information

Patient Name	Anonymous	**Case ID**	LUNG20250813172124
Report Date	2025-08-13 17:21:24	**Image File**	malignant 1.jpg

Diagnostic Analysis

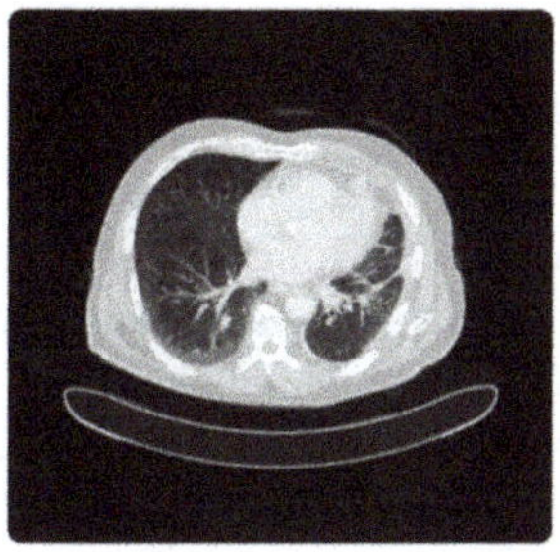

Stage 1: Triage Classification

Finding: Malignant

Model Confidence: 100.00%

The triage model provides an initial assessment of the image for signs of malignancy.

Stage 2: Subtype Classification

Finding: Large Cell Carcinoma

Model Confidence: 99.96%

The subtype model further analyzed the malignant finding to determine the specific type of carcinoma.

Final Conclusion

Malignant - Large Cell Carcinoma

Disclaimer: This report was generated by the HieraLung AI agent. It is intended for use by qualified medical professionals as a clinical decision support tool and is not a substitute for a primary diagnosis. All findings should be correlated with clinical history and other diagnostic tests.

Fig. 7.7 HieraLung diagnostic report (HTML)

7.8 System Architecture and Pipeline

Figure 7.8 shows the HistoLung application flowchart, a linear six-step pipeline: upload image → preprocess → run classification model → get prediction → generate report → display result and offer download. There is no conditional branching; the single CNN produces a direct three-class prediction. Figure 7.9 presents the eight-step HistoLung sequence data flow diagram (User → UI → Agent → Model). The agent preprocesses the image, invokes the CNN, receives class and confidence, compiles the HTML report, and delivers a download link to the user.

7.9 Dataset Used for Development of HistoLung Agent

The HistoLung Agent is trained on the lung subset of the LC25000 (lung and colon cancer histopathological image dataset), a publicly available benchmark dataset created by Borkowski et al. [5] at the James A. Haley Veterans' Hospital, Tampa, Florida, USA. The full LC25000 dataset comprises 25,000 color histopathological images at 768 × 768-pixel resolution across five balanced classes (5000 images each): lung adenocarcinoma, lung squamous cell carcinoma, Lung Benign Tissue, colon adenocarcinoma, and colon benign tissue. For the HistoLung Agent, only the three lung-specific classes are used: lung adenocarcinoma (lung_aca, 5000 images), Lung Benign Tissue (lung_bnt, 5000 images), and lung squamous carcinoma (lung_scc, 5000 images), yielding a total of 15,000 H&E-stained histopathology images. All images are de-identified, HIPAA-compliant, and freely available for research use. The dataset is inherently class-balanced, requiring no additional augmentation for equalization. For the better performance of model, the size of original image increases and makes double for each class, so total of 30,000 images are used for development of HistoLung Agent. For model training, images were resized to 224 × 224 pixels and normalized to [0, 1]. An 80/20 train-validation split was applied with stratified sampling to preserve class balance across partitions.

7.10 CNN Model Architecture and Performance for HistoLung Agent

Table 7.7 presents the CNN architecture used by the HistoLung Agent, which is structurally identical to the HieraLung backbone, three convolutional layers (32 → 64 → 128 filters) with max-pooling after each, followed by flatten, a 512-unit dense layer (carrying the bulk of the ~ 51.5 M parameters), dropout for regularization, and a 3-neuron softmax output layer. The key difference from HieraLung is in the output interpretation: rather than Benign/Malignant/Normal (triage) or cancer subtype categories, HistoLung's output classifies directly into histopathological tissue types,

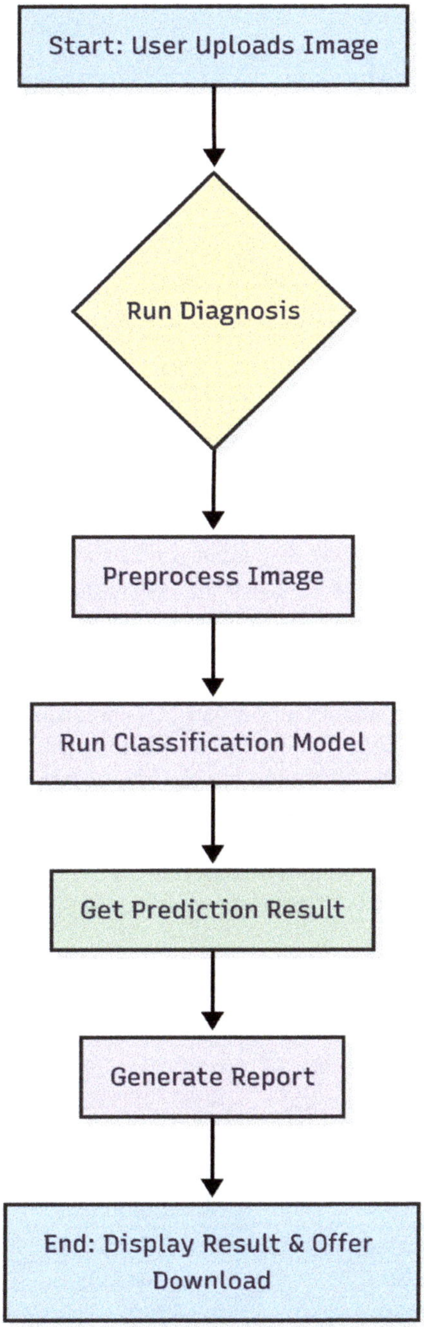

Fig. 7.8 HistoLung application flowchart: linear six-step pipeline from histopathology image upload to diagnostic result display

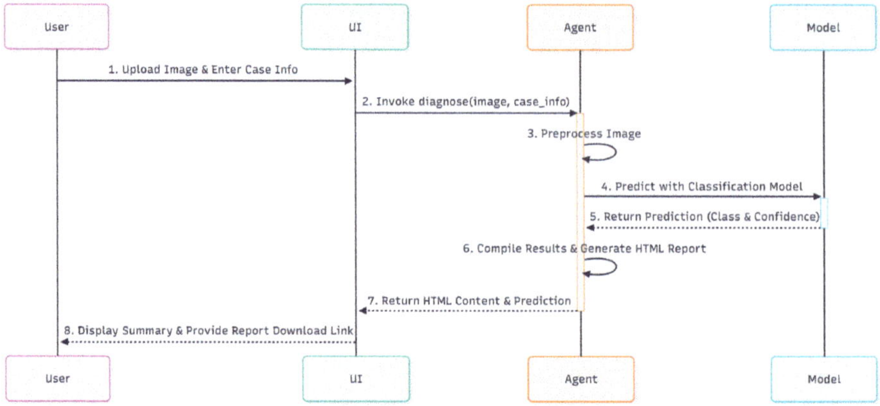

Fig. 7.9 HistoLung 8-step data flow sequence diagram (User, UI, Agent, Model)

lung_aca (adenocarcinoma), lung_bnt (benign tissue), and lung_scc (squamous cell carcinoma). The input is a 224 × 224 px H&E-stained histopathology image rather than a CT scan, and the "Function" column reflects this by describing feature extraction in terms of morphological tissue features rather than radiological features. This architectural sharing across both agents is intentional; it enables a common model framework and simplifies future transfer learning upgrades.

Table 7.8 reports per-class precision, recall, and F1-score for the HistoLung model on both training and validation sets. On training data, performance is near-perfect across all three classes (Macro F1: 0.9865), with Lung Benign Tissue achieving 0.9964 F1 and even the weakest class (SCC) at 0.9831. On validation, performance drops to a Macro F1 of 0.9122 (91.15% accuracy), with a notable gap: Benign tissue remains strong (F1 0.9797), but adenocarcinoma drops to 0.8741 F1 (high recall 0.9215 but lower precision 0.8313, meaning that it over-predicts ACA) and

Table 7.7 CNN_LC_Histo_Classifier architecture, total trainable parameters: 51,475,523

Layer	Output shape	Parameters	Function
conv2d (Conv2D)	(None, 224, 224, 32)	896	Feature extraction from H&E image
max_pooling2d	(None, 112, 112, 32)	0	Spatial downsampling (2 × 2)
conv2d_1	(None, 112, 112, 64)	18,496	Intermediate tissue feature maps
max_pooling2d_1	(None, 56, 56, 64)	0	Spatial downsampling (2 × 2)
conv2d_2	(None, 56, 56, 128)	73,856	High-level morphological features
max_pooling2d_2	(None, 28, 28, 128)	0	Final downsampling
Flatten	(None, 100,352)	0	3D → 1D feature vector
dense (Dense)	(None, 512)	51,380,736	Fully connected classification head
Dropout	(None, 512)	0	Regularization
dense_1	(None, 3)	1,539	Output: lung_aca/lung_bnt/lung_scc

Table 7.8 CNN_LC_Histo_Classifier training and validation report

Class	Precision	Recall	F1	Dataset
Lung adenocarcinoma (ACA)	0.9642	0.9965	0.9801	Training
Lung Benign Tissue (BNT)	0.9997	0.9931	0.9964	Training
Lung squamous cell carc. (SCC)	0.9967	0.9699	0.9831	Training
Macro avg.	0.9869	0.9865	0.9865	Training
Lung adenocarcinoma (ACA)	0.8313	0.9215	0.8741	Validation
Lung benign tissue (BNT)	0.9969	0.9630	0.9797	Validation
Lung squamous cell carc. (SCC)	0.9184	0.8500	0.8829	Validation
Macro avg.	0.9155	0.9115	0.9122	Validation

SCC falls to 0.8829 F1 (lower recall 0.8500, meaning that some SCC cases are misclassified). The training-to-validation gap (~ 7.4% F1 drop) indicates moderate overfitting, and the ACA-SCC confusion pattern is clinically expected since these two NSCLC subtypes can share overlapping morphological features on H&E staining.

7.11 User Interface of HieraLung Agent

7.11.1 Landing Screen

Figure 7.10 shows the HistoLung landing screen. The sidebar provides Case Information and an Upload Histopathology Image widget. The main panel presents dual column "Uploaded Image" and "Diagnostic Summary" placeholders with upload prompts.

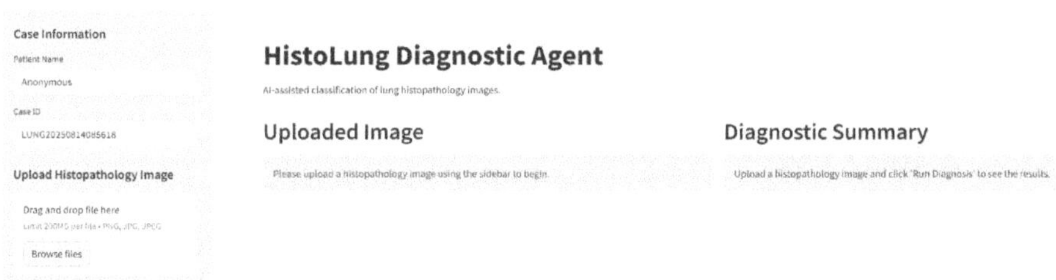

Fig. 7.10 HistoLung landing screen

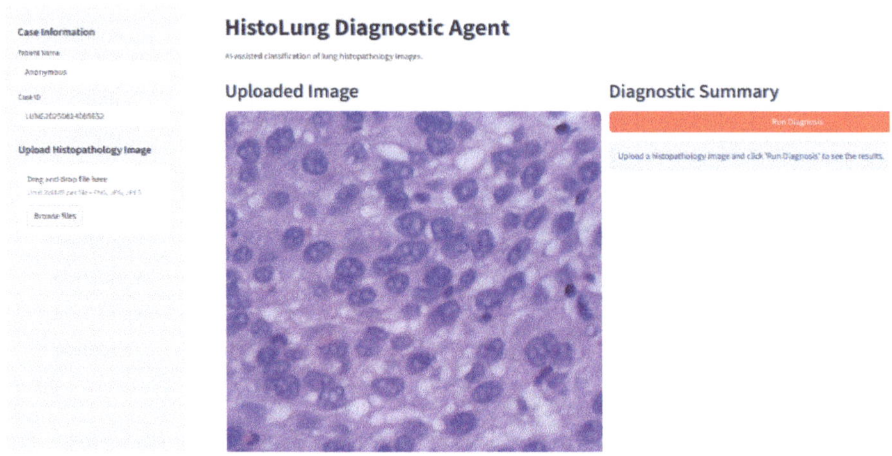

Fig. 7.11 HistoLung post-upload state

7.11.2 Post-upload State

Figure 7.11 shows the interface after uploading H&E image. The left column renders the H&E slide showing densely packed tumor cells with pleomorphic nuclear morphology. A red "Run Diagnosis" button appears in the right column.

7.11.3 Post-prediction Results

Figure 7.12 shows the diagnostic summary post-analysis: Stage 1 finding: lung squamous cell carcinoma (SCC), confidence: 58.81%. The moderate confidence score appropriately signals the need for pathologist confirmation.

7.11.4 Report Download State

Figure 7.13 captures the browser download notification confirming "HistoLung_Report_LUNG20250814085754.html" downloaded successfully. The "Download Full Report (HTML)" button highlighted in red indicates that it was activated.

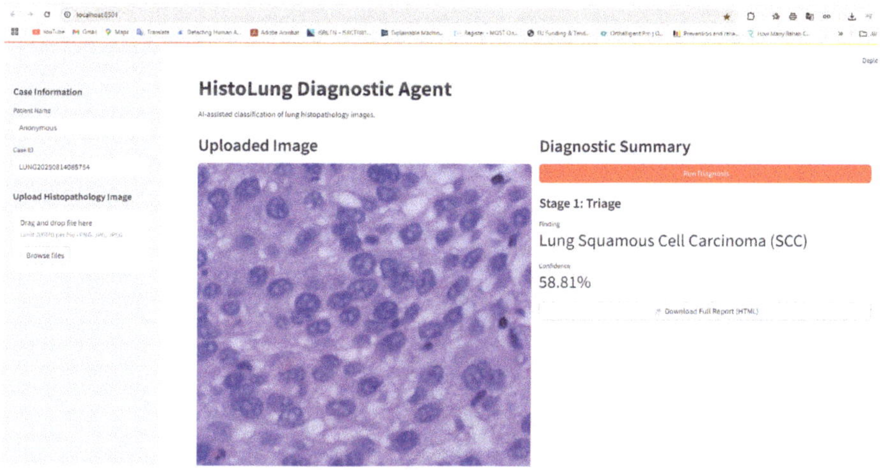

Fig. 7.12 HistoLung post-diagnosis results

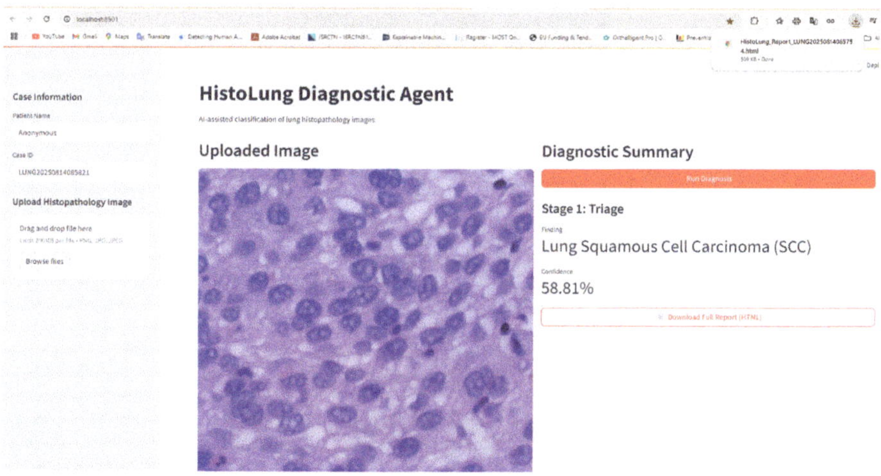

Fig. 7.13 HistoLung report download state

7.12 Generated HistoLung Report

Figure 7.14 presents the HTML report for Case ID LUNG20250814085754. Sections: (1) Patient and Case Information; (2) Diagnostic Analysis with H&E slide image; (3) Stage 1: Triage Classification, Lung Squamous Cell Carcinoma (SCC), Model Confidence: 58.81%; (4) Final Conclusion: Lung Squamous Cell Carcinoma (SCC); (5) Disclaimer.

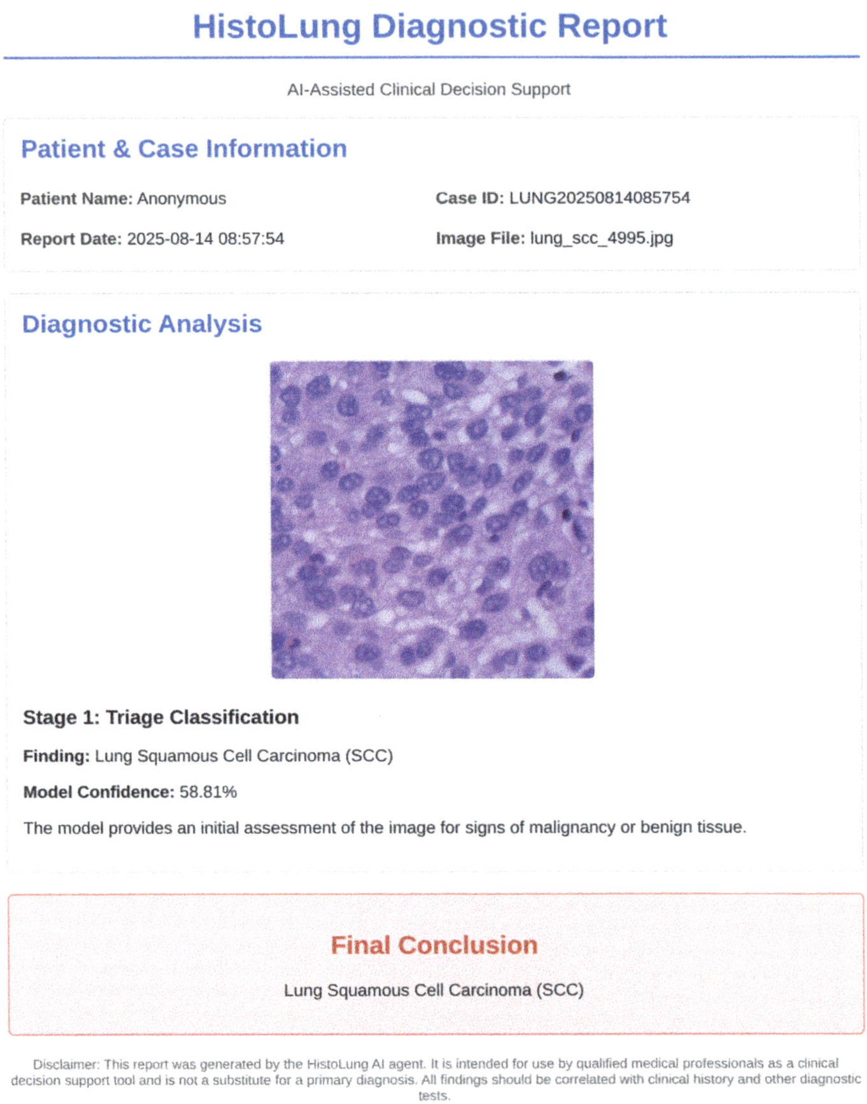

HistoLung Diagnostic Report

AI-Assisted Clinical Decision Support

Patient & Case Information

Patient Name: Anonymous

Case ID: LUNG20250814085754

Report Date: 2025-08-14 08:57:54

Image File: lung_scc_4995.jpg

Diagnostic Analysis

Stage 1: Triage Classification

Finding: Lung Squamous Cell Carcinoma (SCC)

Model Confidence: 58.81%

The model provides an initial assessment of the image for signs of malignancy or benign tissue.

Final Conclusion

Lung Squamous Cell Carcinoma (SCC)

Disclaimer: This report was generated by the HistoLung AI agent. It is intended for use by qualified medical professionals as a clinical decision support tool and is not a substitute for a primary diagnosis. All findings should be correlated with clinical history and other diagnostic tests.

Fig. 7.14 HistoLung diagnostic report (HTML)

7.13 Summary

HieraLung and HistoLung address two distinct and complementary stages of the imaging-based lung cancer diagnostic pathway. HieraLung provides radiological screening from CT scans through a clinically logical hierarchical pipeline; HistoLung provides pathological confirmation from H&E tissue slides through a direct single-model pipeline. Their architecturally shared CNN backbone enables parallel deployment from a common model framework, simplifying maintenance and future transfer learning upgrades. Both agents are designed to function as standalone clinical decision-support tools and as constituent components of the MLCA Agent (Chapter 8), which orchestrates their outputs alongside the LCRP Agent risk score and a Generative AI synthesis layer to produce a holistic multi-modal diagnostic report.

References

1. Ardila, D., Kiraly, A. P., Bharadwaj, S., Choi, B., Reicher, J. J., Peng, L., Tse, D., Etemadi, M., Ye, W., Corrado, G., Naidich, D. P., & Shetty, S. (2019). End-to-end lung cancer screening with three-dimensional deep learning on low-dose chest computed tomography. *Nature Medicine, 25*(6), 954–961.
2. Alyasriy, H., & Al-Huseiny, M. (2020). *The IQ-OTHNCCD lung cancer dataset. Mendeley data.*
3. Hany, M. (2020). *Chest CT-scan images dataset CT-scan images with different types of chest cancer*. Weblink: https://www.kaggle.com/datasets/mohamedhanyyy/chest-ctscan-images. Last Access: September 2025.
4. Coudray, N., Ocampo, P. S., Sakellaropoulos, T., Narula, N., Snuderl, M., Fenyö, D., Moreira, A. L., Razavian, N., & Tsirigos, A. (2018). Classification and mutation prediction from non–small cell lung cancer histopathology images using deep learning. *Nature Medicine, 24*(10), 1559–1567.
5. Borkowski, A. A., Bui, M. M., Thomas, L. B., Wilson, C. P., DeLand, L. A., & Mastorides, S. M. (2019). Lung and colon cancer histopathological image dataset (lc25000). arXiv preprint arXiv:1912.12142

Chapter 8
The Multi-modal Lung Cancer Assessment (MLCA) Agent

This chapter presents the Multi-modal Lung Cancer Assessment (MLCA) Agent, the apex of the AI diagnostic ecosystem documented in this book. The MLCA Agent orchestrates the LCRP Agent (Chap. 6), HieraLung Agent (Chap. 7A), and HistoLung Agent (Chap. 7B) in parallel and then synthesizes all three streams of specialist AI analysis using a large language model (e.g., Ollama, google Gemini, OpenAI GPT-4o) to produce a single holistic, structured clinical report. In doing so, it emulates the integrative reasoning of a Multidisciplinary Team (MDT) tumor board—the gold standard for lung cancer diagnosis and treatment planning [1].

8.1 Introduction and Clinical Motivation

Single-modality AI tools, however accurate, can only address one dimension of the diagnostic question. Clinical risk assessment, CT imaging, and histopathology each provide partial evidence; definitive diagnostic confidence requires their synthesis [2]. The MLCA Agent addresses this challenge through a two-stage architecture: Stage 1 runs three parallel specialized AI models; Stage 2 uses a Generative AI LLM to perform concordance analysis, risk stratification, and clinical recommendation generation tasks that mirror the cognitive work of an MDT tumor board [3].

8.2 System Architecture

Figure 8.1 presents the high-level system architecture. Three input modalities (patient clinical data CSV, CT scan image, histopathology image) flow through three specialized analysis modules, converge at a Generative AI synthesis stage, and produce

S. Shah and R. Thanki, *Artificial Intelligence for Early Detection and Diagnosis of Lung Cancer*, Signals and Communication Technology,
https://doi.org/10.1007/978-3-032-29615-3_8

a comprehensive diagnostic report (HTML). AI models are housed as local files (joblib, h5); LLM inference is performed via an external API call.

Figure 8.2 shows internal backend component interactions. The Streamlit Server Logic dispatches data to three agents (LCRP, HieraLung, HistoLung), aggregates their results, and passes them to the ReportGeneration Module, which calls the external Generative AI API and returns the holistic report.

Figure 8.3 shows the deployment architecture: clinician browser accesses via HTTPS; Python backend on Cloud Server/VM loads three local model file sets and makes external API calls to Generative AI API.

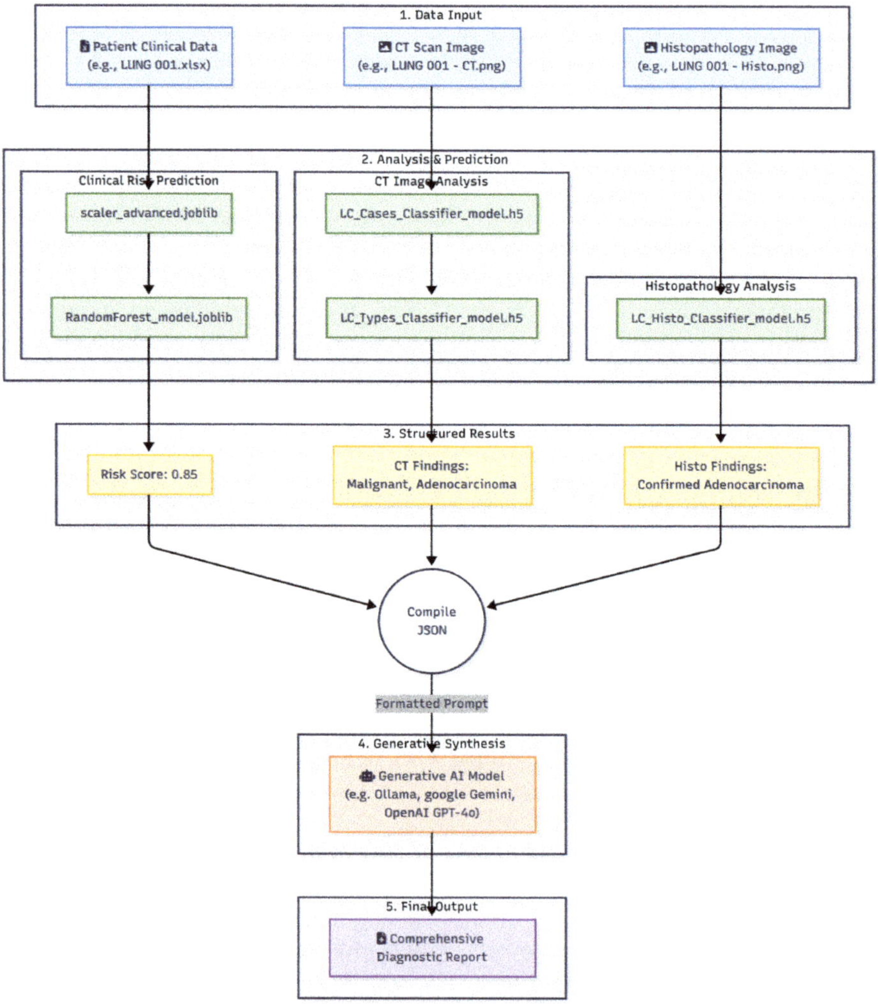

Fig. 8.1 MLCA agent system architecture: three parallel input modalities → three specialized AI modules → generative AI synthesis → comprehensive diagnostic report

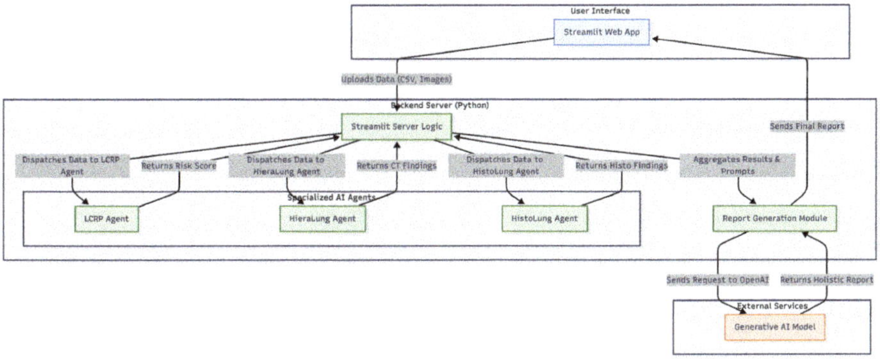

Fig. 8.2 MLCA agent application-level diagram. Streamlit server logic orchestrates LCRP, HieraLung, HistoLung agents and report generation module (external generative AI API)

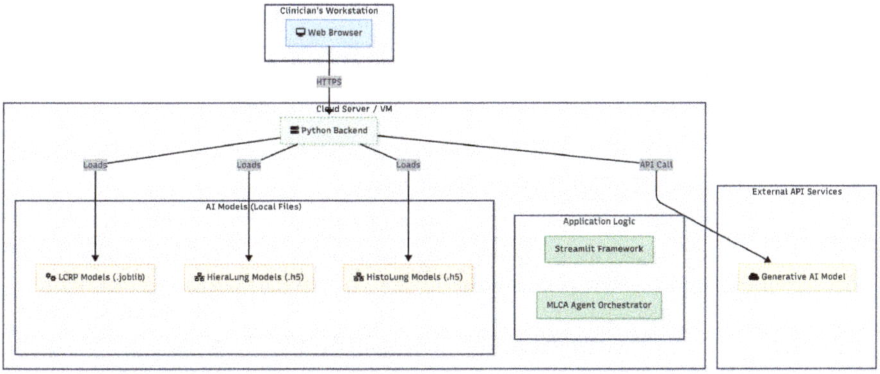

Fig. 8.3 MLCA agent deployment: HTTPS → Python backend on Cloud/VM → local AI model files (LCRP.joblib; HieraLung.h5; HistoLung.h5) + external generative AI API

8.3 Class Diagram for Object-Oriented Design

Figure 8.4 presents the UML class diagram. Streamlit App orchestrates four downstream classes via "uses" relationships: LCRP Agent, HieraLung Agent, HistoLung Agent, and ReportGenerator. ReportGenerator uses Generative AI Client to interface with the LLM API.

Table 8.1 expands the UML class diagram (as shown in Fig. 8.4) into a structured component reference, documenting the key attributes, primary methods, and architectural roles of all six classes in the MLCA Agent object model. The Streamlit App class serves as the top-level orchestrator, collecting patient inputs and delegating analysis to three specialist agent classes (LCRP Agent, HieraLung Agent, HistoLung Agent), each encapsulating its respective AI model and inference logic. The ReportGenerator class aggregates Stage 1 outputs and interfaces with the Generative AI

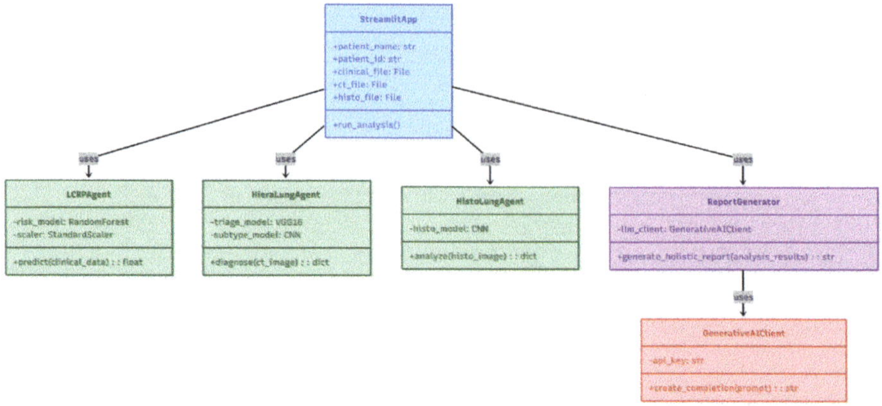

Fig. 8.4 MLCA agent UML class diagram. Streamlit App orchestrates LCRP Agent, HieraLung Agent, HistoLung agent, and report generator (which uses generative AI client)

Client class, which manages the external LLM provider like Ollama, Google Gemini OpenAI GPT-4o API connection for holistic report synthesis.

Table 8.1 All six classes in the MLCA agent object model

Class	Key attributes	Primary method	Architectural role
Streamlit App	patient_name, patient_id, clinical_file, ct_file, histo_file	run_analysis()	Top-level orchestrator; collects input and delegates to sub-agents
LCRP Agent	risk_model: Random forest, scaler: StandardScaler	predict(clinical_data): float	Processes CSV; returns clinical risk score
HieraLung Agent	triage_model: VGG16, subtype_model: CNN	diagnose(ct_image): dict	Hierarchical CT triage and conditional subtype classification
HistoLung Agent	histo_model: CNN	analyze(histo_image): dict	Classifies H&E slide into ACA/BNT/SCC
ReportGenerator	llm_client: Generative AI Client	generate_holistic_report(results): str	Aggregates Stage 1 results; generates LLM narrative
Generative AI Client	api_key: str	create_completion(prompt): str	External LLM API interface

8.4 Data Flow and Sequence Diagrams

Figure 8.5 illustrates how data move through both pipeline stages. Three raw inputs are processed in parallel by their respective models, producing Risk Score, CT Triage and Subtype Findings, and Histopathology Finding. All outputs are compiled into a structured JSON prompt sent to the Generative AI Model, which produces the Comprehensive Diagnostic Report.

Figure 8.6 presents the 12-step sequence diagram showing interactions between Clinician, Streamlit App, LCRP Agent, HieraLung Agent, HistoLung Agent, Report Generator, and Generative AI API during a full diagnostic session.

Table 8.2 provides the complete 12-step interaction flow derived from the sequence diagram (as shown in Fig. 8.6), detailing each message exchange between the Clinician, Streamlit App, specialist agents, Report Generator, and Generative AI API during a full diagnostic session. Steps 1–7 cover the data upload and parallel specialist agent analysis phase: The clinician uploads three input files, and the Streamlit App

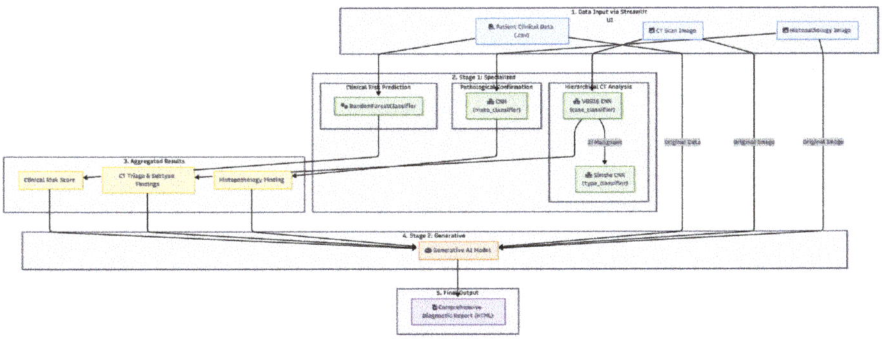

Fig. 8.5 MLCA agent data flow: three parallel Stage 1 pipelines converge into a JSON prompt for Generative AI synthesis, producing the comprehensive diagnostic report

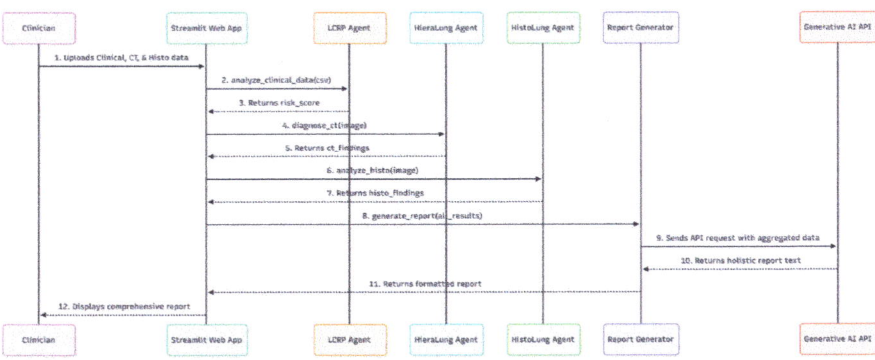

Fig. 8.6 MLCA agent 12-step sequence diagram. Steps 1–7: data upload and parallel specialist agent analysis. Steps 8–12: LLM synthesis and report delivery

Table 8.2 Detailed 12-step interaction flow for the MLCA agent

Step	Sender	Receiver	Message/action
1	Clinician	Streamlit App	Uploads clinical CSV, CT scan, and histopathology image
2	Streamlit App	LCRP Agent	analyze_clinical_data(csv) dispatches clinical data
3	LCRP Agent	Streamlit App	Returns risk_score (e.g., 96.00%)
4	Streamlit App	HieraLung Agent	diagnose_ct(image) dispatches CT image
5	HieraLung Agent	Streamlit App	Returns ct_findings {triage, subtype, confidence}
6	Streamlit App	HistoLung Agent	analyze_histo(image) dispatches H&E slide
7	HistoLung Agent	Streamlit App	Returns histo_findings {class, confidence}
8	Streamlit App	Report Generator	generate_report(all_results) aggregates Stage 1 outputs
9	Report Generator	Generative AI API	Sends structured JSON prompt and patient data
10	Generative AI API	Report Generator	Returns holistic report text (narrative synthesis)
11	Report Generator	Streamlit App	Returns formatted HTML report content
12	Streamlit App	Clinician	Displays comprehensive report with Download Full Report link

dispatches each to its respective agent (LCRP, HieraLung, HistoLung), collecting risk scores, CT findings, and histopathology results. Steps 8–12 cover the LLM synthesis and report delivery phase: the Report Generator aggregates all Stage 1 outputs, sends a structured JSON prompt to the OpenAI GPT-4o API, receives the holistic narrative synthesis, formats the HTML report, and delivers it to the clinician for download.

8.5 Two-Stage Processing Pipeline

This section covers the two-stage pipeline concept separating specialized AI inference (Stage 1) from integrative LLM reasoning (Stage 2), the parallel execution of three specialist agents, the five cognitive synthesis tasks performed by Generative AI model such as GPT-4o, the MDT tumor board analogy, and a forward reference to Tables 8.3 and 8.4 for the detailed breakdowns.

Table 8.3 Three parallel Stage 1 specialized analysis pipelines

Pipeline	Input	AI model(s)	Output	Agent (chapter)
Clinical risk prediction	Patient clinical CSV	Random forest + StandardScaler (.joblib)	Risk score 0–1	LCRP Agent (Chap. 6)
CT radiological analysis	CT scan image (.jpg/.png)	VGG16 CNN (triage) + Simple CNN (subtype)	Malignancy + subtype + confidence	HieraLung Agent (Chap. 7A)
Histopathology Analysis	H&E biopsy slide (.jpg/.png)	Simple CNN—3-class histo classifier	ACA/SCC/BNT + confidence	HistoLung Agent (Chap. 7B)

Table 8.4 Five core tasks performed by the generative AI model in Stage 2 of the MLCA Agent

LLM task	Description	Example output
Concordance/discordance analysis	Cross-compare CT, histopathology, and clinical risk findings for agreement or conflict	High concordance: CT = SCC, Histo = SCC, Risk = 96% → strengthens diagnostic confidence
Summary of findings	Translate each modality's technical outputs into a clinical narrative paragraph	Plain-language summaries for clinical data, CT findings, and histopathology results
Overall risk stratification	Integrate all modalities into a unified clinical impression with risk level	High risk, concordant malignant findings across imaging and pathology
Clinical recommendations	Suggest evidence-based next steps aligned with standard oncological practice	PET/CT, bronchoscopy, MDT meeting, PD-L1 expression analysis, staging
Human-readable report	Format synthesized findings into a structured professional medical report	Downloadable HTML report with sections: summary, concordance, risk, recommendations, disclaimer

8.5.1 Stage 1: Parallel Specialized AI Analysis

Table 8.3 summarizes the three parallel specialized analysis pipelines that constitute Stage 1 of the MLCA Agent. Each pipeline operates independently on a distinct input modality: clinical CSV data processed by the LCRP Agent (Chap. 6) using a Random Forest classifier with StandardScaler preprocessing, CT scan images analyzed by the HieraLung Agent (Chap. 7A) through a two-model hierarchical CNN pipeline (VGG16 triage followed by subtype CNN), and H&E-stained histopathology slides classified by the HistoLung Agent (Chap. 7B) using a single three-class CNN. The three pipelines execute in parallel within the Streamlit application, and their outputs, a clinical risk score, CT-derived malignancy and subtype findings with confidence scores, and a histopathological tissue classification with confidence are subsequently aggregated for Stage 2 synthesis.

8.5.2 *Stage 2: Generative AI Synthesis*

Stage 2 is the defining innovation of the MLCA Agent. The outputs from Stage 1 are compiled into a structured JSON prompt and passed to any Generative AI API, here used OpenAI GPT-4o. The LLM performs five cognitive tasks [4]: concordance/discordance analysis, summary of findings, overall risk stratification, clinical recommendations, and human-readable report generation. Table 8.4 details the five discrete cognitive tasks performed by the Generative AI model (OpenAI GPT-4o) during Stage 2 synthesis.

These tasks range from cross-comparing the outputs of all three Stage 1 agents for concordance or discordance, through translating technical model outputs into plain-language clinical narratives, to generating an overall risk stratification and evidence-based clinical recommendations. The final task produces a structured, human-readable HTML report suitable for clinical documentation and MDT referral.

8.6 User Interface of MLCA Agent

This section presents MLCA Agent's Streamlit-based clinical interface at each stage of a complete diagnostic session. The interface follows a progressive workflow: the landing screen (Sect. 8.6.1) provides patient identification fields and three separate file upload widgets for the clinical CSV, CT scan, and histopathology image; the post-upload state (Sect. 8.6.2) confirms all three files are loaded and activates the analysis trigger; the post-analysis view (Sect. 8.6.3) displays the three-panel Stage 1 results showing clinical risk score, CT findings, and histopathology classification side by side; and the holistic report view (Sect. 8.6.4) renders the full LLM-generated narrative report in line with a download option. Together, these screenshots document the end-to-end clinician experience from data input through multi-modal AI analysis to actionable diagnostic output.

8.6.1 *Landing Screen*

Figure 8.7 shows the MLCA Agent landing screen. The left sidebar presents Patient Name (John Doe), Patient ID (P123456), and three separate file upload widgets (Clinical CSV, CT scan PNG/JPG, Histopathology PNG/JPG) plus the "Generate Holistic Report" button.

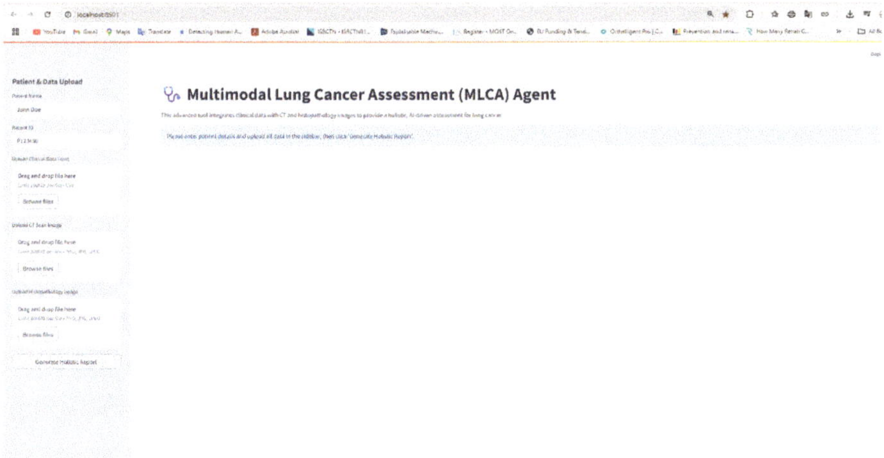

Fig. 8.7 MLCA Agent landing screen

8.6.2 Post-Upload State, All Three Files Loaded

Figure 8.8 shows all three input files confirmed in the sidebar: Patient Data (ID with P123456) LUNG 001 (CSV), CT LUNG 001.jpg, Histo LUNG 001.jpg. The "Generate Holistic Report" button is now active.

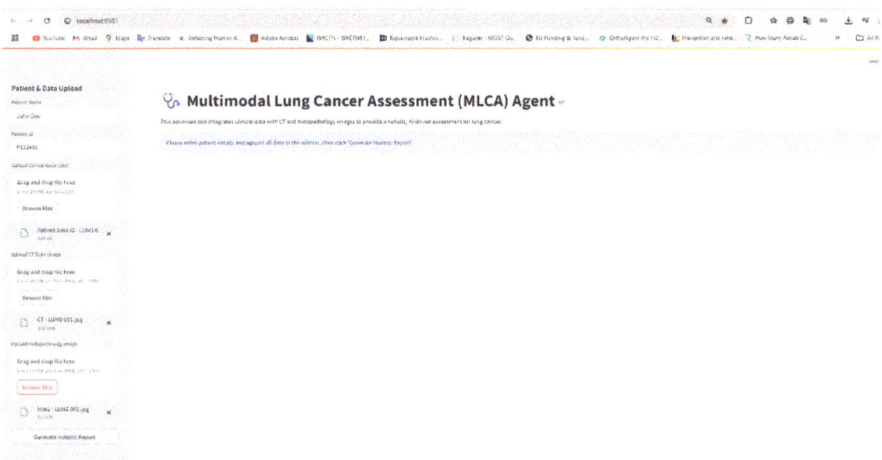

Fig. 8.8 MLCA Agent post-upload state

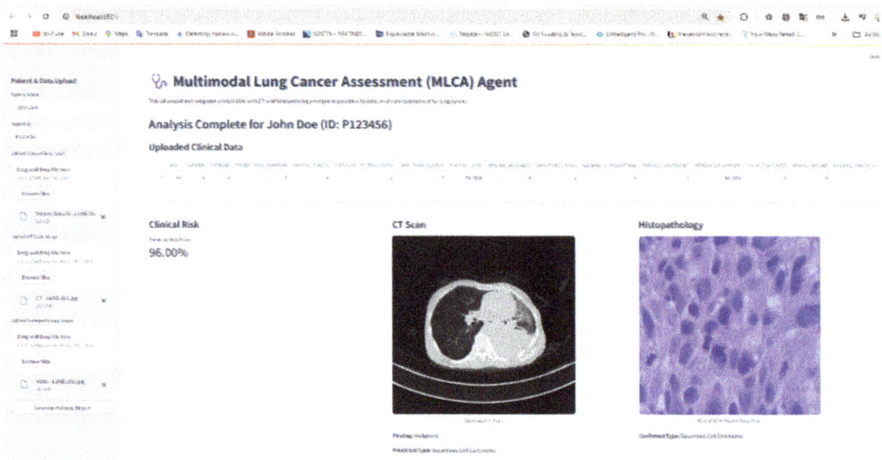

Fig. 8.9 MLCA Agent three-panel analysis results

8.6.3 Post-Analysis Results 1 (Three AI Analysis)

Figure 8.9 shows the analysis results for Patient John Doe (ID: P123456). The panel displays: (1) Uploaded Clinical Data table (all 17 features extracted from CSV); (2) Three-panel results, Clinical Risk: 96.00%; CT scan: Malignant, SCC; Histopathology: Squamous Cell Carcinoma.

8.6.4 Post-Analysis Results 2 (Holistic AI Report)

Figure 8.10 presents the LLM-generated "Holistic AI-Generated Report" displayed inline in the application. Five sections are visible: (1) Summary of Findings; (2) Concordance/Discordance Analysis; (3) Overall Assessment and Risk Stratification; (4) Clinical Recommendations, Immediate Staging (Chest X-ray, Full Body CT, PET/CT, Bronchoscopy, Brain MRI), MDT Meeting, Biomarker Analysis (PD-L1); (5) Disclaimer. A "Download Full Report (HTML)" button appears below.

8.7 Generated Report of Multi-modal Lung Cancer Analysis Report

Figure 8.11 presents the downloaded HTML report for Patient John Doe (ID: P123456). The report contains five sections: (1) Patient and Case Information: comprehensive metadata and all 17 clinical parameters; (2) Diagnostic Analysis:

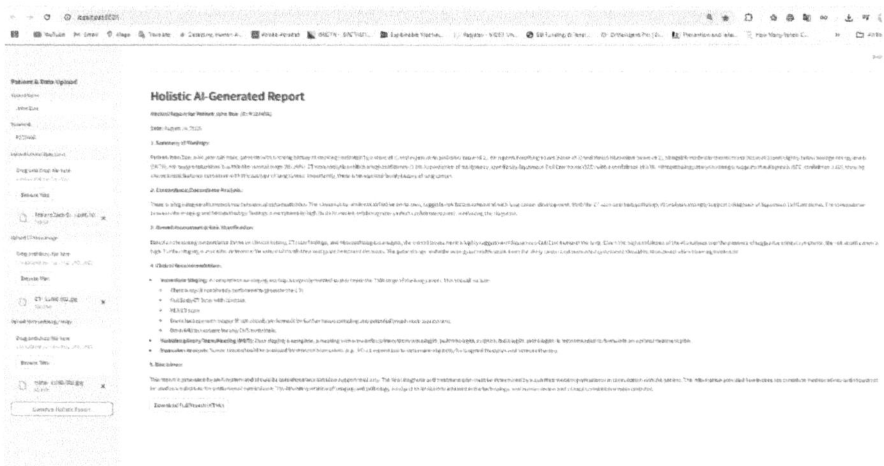

Fig. 8.10 MLCA Agent holistic AI-generated report

CT and H&E images with three result callout blocks (Stage 1 CT Triage: Malignant 100%; Stage 2 CT Subtype: SCC 97.90%; Histopathology: SCC 99.87%); (3) Final Conclusion: Malignant (Squamous Cell Carcinoma); (4) Holistic AI-Generated Report, full LLM narrative with clinical data analysis, CT analysis, histopathology analysis, concordance analysis, unified clinical impression, risk level, clinical recommendations, and treatment considerations; (5) Disclaimer.

8.8 Illustrative Case Results and Cross-Modality Concordance

Table 8.5 presents the end-to-end results of the MLCA Agent for the illustrative case of Patient John Doe (ID: P123456l). The table traces the diagnostic output through each stage of the pipeline: LCRP Agent clinical risk prediction (96.00%), HieraLung Agent CT triage (Malignant, 100.00% confidence) and subtype classification (Squamous Cell Carcinoma, 97.90% confidence), and HistoLung Agent histopathological analysis (SCC, 99.87% confidence).

The cross-modality concordance row highlights that all three independent modalities unanimously support a Malignant, Squamous Cell Carcinoma diagnosis, enabling the GPT-4o synthesis layer to produce an unambiguous holistic report with high clinical confidence. This concordance pattern represents the ideal operational scenario for the MLCA Agent, where converging multi-modal evidence strengthens the diagnostic conclusion beyond what any single modality could achieve alone.

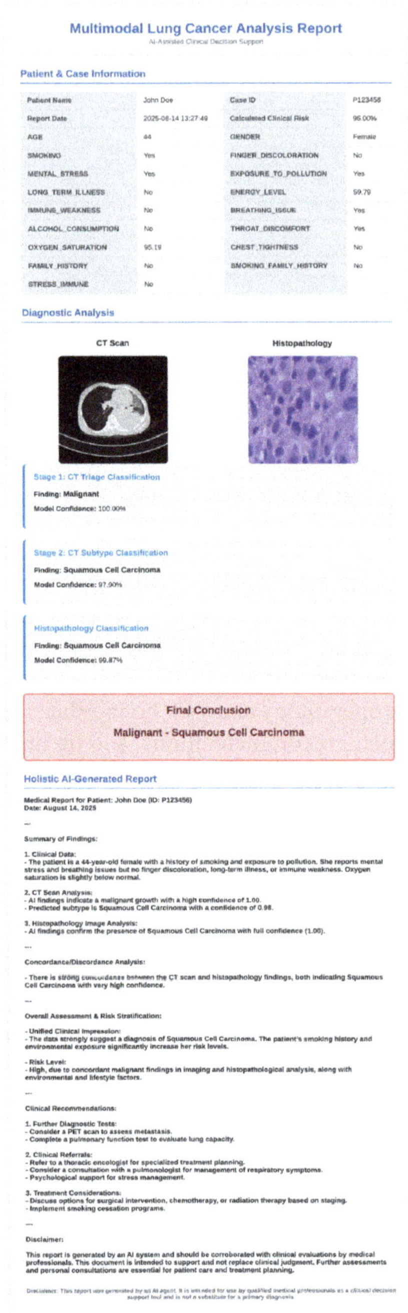

Fig. 8.11 MLCA Agent downloaded HTML report

Table 8.5 Illustrative case results

Stage	Model/agent	Result	Interpretation
Clinical risk	LCRP Agent (Random Forest)	96.00%	Very high risk: smoking, pollution, breathing issues, throat discomfort all flagged
CT Stage 1 (triage)	HieraLung Agent (VGG16)	Malignant (100.00%)	Maximum confidence; pipeline advances to subtype model
CT Stage 2 (subtype)	HieraLung Agent (CNN)	SCC (97.90%)	Squamous Cell Carcinoma confirmed from CT morphological features
Histopathology	HistoLung Agent (CNN)	SCC (99.87%)	H&E slide independently confirms SCC with near-perfect confidence
Cross-modality concordance	LLM Analysis	HIGH	All three modalities concordantly support Malignant, SCC: no conflict
Conclusion	GPT-4o Synthesis	Malignant, SCC	Holistic report: immediate staging workup, MDT, PD-L1 biomarker recommended

8.9 Clinical Value, Limitations, and Future Directions

The MLCA Agent achieves three clinical value propositions beyond any single-modality agent: (1) Cross-modality concordance analysis, determining whether imaging, pathology, and clinical data agree; (2) Conflict flagging, identifying discordant findings that require clinical caution; and (3) Evidence-based clinical recommendations, generating next-step guidance aligned with oncological standards [5]. By emulating MDT reasoning in software, the MLCA Agent has the potential to improve diagnostic efficiency in under-resourced settings where weekly tumor boards are unavailable or delayed.

Key limitations include: LLM output stochasticity (requiring temperature control in production); the MLCA inheriting the performance bounds of its constituent models; and the OpenAI API dependency raising data governance concerns in regulated healthcare environments. Future development priorities include: (a) local open-weight LLM deployment (e.g., Llama 3, Mistral) for data sovereignty compliance [6]; (b) genomic and liquid biopsy data stream integration; and (c) prospective clinical validation against confirmed MDT outcomes.

8.10 Summary

The Multi-modal Lung Cancer Assessment (MLCA) Agent is a two-stage artificial intelligence diagnostic system that integrates clinical risk prediction, hierarchical CT analysis, and histopathology classification in parallel. After these assessments, Generative AI synthesis produces a comprehensive, clinically actionable diagnostic report. Its object-oriented architecture comprises six core components, supported by diagrams and tables illustrating its modular design and workflow. The MLCA Agent delivers key clinical value by performing multi-modal concordance analysis, flagging conflicts among findings, and providing evidence-based clinical recommendations, which together enhance the reliability and actionability of diagnoses. A case study highlighted the agent's effectiveness by demonstrating consistent diagnosis of squamous cell carcinoma (SCC) across all modalities. Nonetheless, limitations remain, including reliance on constituent models, variability in large language model outputs, and dependency on external APIs. Future advancements aim to deploy local LLMs, integrate genomic and liquid biopsy data streams, and undertake clinical validation studies to reinforce the system's performance and reliability.

References

1. Detterbeck, F. C., Boffa, D. J., Kim, A. W., & Tanoue, L. T. (2017). The eighth edition lung cancer stage classification. *Chest, 151*(1), 193–203.
2. Acosta, J. N., Falcone, G. J., Rajpurkar, P., & Topol, E. J. (2022). Multimodal biomedical AI. *Nature Medicine, 28*(9), 1773–1784.
3. Topol, E. J. (2019). High-performance medicine: The convergence of human and artificial intelligence. *Nature Medicine, 25*(1), 44–56.
4. Singhal, K., Azizi, S., Tu, T., Mahdavi, S. S., Wei, J., Chung, H. W., Scales, N., Tanwani, A., Cole-Lewis, H., Pfohl, S., Payne, P., & Natarajan, V. (2023). Large language models encode clinical knowledge. *Nature, 620*(7972), 172-180.
5. Postmus, P. E., Kerr, K. M., Oudkerk, M., Senan, S., Waller, D. A., Vansteenkiste, J., Escriu, C., Peters, S., & ESMO Guidelines Committee. (2017). Early and locally advanced non-small-cell lung cancer (NSCLC): ESMO Clinical Practice Guidelines for diagnosis, treatment and follow-up. *Annals of Oncology, 28,* iv1–iv21.
6. Rajpurkar, P., Chen, E., Banerjee, O., & Topol, E. J. (2022). AI in health and medicine. *Nature Medicine, 28*(1), 31–38.

Index

A
Adenocarcinoma, 4, 8, 14, 26, 37, 38, 56, 107, 111–114, 120
AI-assisted radiology, 61
Algorithmic bias, 62
ALK, 5, 8, 28, 38, 48, 65, 66, 81
Artificial Intelligence (AI), 43, 55, 65, 107

B
Biomarker discovery, 67, 71, 69, 80, 93
Biopsy, 8, 9, 21, 23, 27–32, 34, 38, 57, 60, 62, 93, 116, 133, 139, 140
BorderlineSMOTE, 68, 69, 92

C
Cancer, 1, 14–21, 23–40, 44, 45, 51, 65, 71, 72, 77, 81, 82, 90, 98, 100, 107, 118
Cancer classification, 6, 66
Cancer diagnosis, 2, 7
Cancer prevention, 2, 3, 18–20
Carcinogens, 2, 3, 16–19, 21, 99
Checkpoint inhibitors, 10, 39
Chemotherapy, 2, 9–11, 15, 21, 25, 26, 31–34, 36–40, 80
Chest CT-scan dataset, 110, 111
Class balancing, 118
Clinical decision support, 44, 45, 50, 51, 60, 86, 125
Computer-Aided Diagnosis (CAD), 46
Computer Vision (CV), 43–45, 51, 72, 87
Concordance analysis, 127, 137, 139, 140
Contrastive learning, 58
Convolutional Neural Network (CNN), 44–47, 55, 59, 107, 111, 116, 118, 130, 133
Cox proportional, 66, 71, 78, 79, 90
Cross-modality concordance, 137, 139
CT scan classification, 107

D
Deep Learning (DL), 43–48, 50, 51, 61, 66, 76
Diagnostic report, 105, 116, 125, 140
Drug repurposing, 67, 69, 71, 72, 85

E
EGFR, 5, 8, 10, 17, 28, 37, 38, 48, 50, 65, 66, 80, 81, 83, 94
Electronic Health Records (EHR), 47, 51, 56–58, 62, 103, 105
Explainable AI (XAI), 60, 62

F
Federated Learning (FL), 48, 58, 59
Foundation models, 56, 62

G
Gene Expression Omnibus (GEO), 67, 68, 92, 93
Gene expression profiling, 66
Generative AI, 44, 51, 61, 105, 125, 127–132, 134, 140
GPT-4o, 127, 130, 132, 134, 137, 139

S. Shah and R. Thanki, *Artificial Intelligence for Early Detection and Diagnosis of Lung Cancer*, Signals and Communication Technology,
https://doi.org/10.1007/978-3-032-29615-3

Grad-CAM, 60
Gradient boosting, 76, 98–100

H
Hazards, 18, 66, 71, 79, 90
H&E staining, 121
HieraLung, 107, 108, 113, 128, 129, 132
Hierarchical classification, 107
Histology, 6, 81
HistoLung, 107, 127–133, 137, 139
Histopathology, 43, 44, 48, 50, 51, 66, 75, 105, 107, 127, 131–134, 137, 139, 140
Holistic diagnostic report, 105
HTML report, 97, 98, 103, 108, 115, 118, 123, 132–134, 136, 138

I
Immunotherapy, 2, 8, 10, 15, 21, 23, 25, 33–35, 39, 40, 65, 82, 85, 86, 91, 93
IQ-OTH/NCCD dataset, 110, 111

K
Kaplan–Meier (KM), 66, 70, 76–79, 93
KRAS, 5, 28, 38, 66, 80, 81, 94

L
Large cell carcinoma, 14, 26, 107, 111–114, 116
Large Language Model (LLM), 61, 62, 93, 127–134, 136, 137, 139, 140
LC25000 dataset, 118
LCRP agent, 97–99, 101–105, 125, 127, 129–133, 137, 139
Liquid biopsy, 57, 60, 62, 93, 139, 140
Lobectomy, 33, 34
Low-Dose CT screening, 29
LungAI-Dx, 65
Lung anatomy, 12
Lung cancer, 1, 23, 43, 55, 65, 66, 97, 99, 100, 102, 107, 116, 124, 127, 136
Lung Cancer Risk Prediction (LCRP), 97, 128, 129
Lung Cancer Screening (LCS), 30, 31, 43, 48, 51, 55, 56, 60, 62
Lung cancer staging, 23, 29, 31

M
Machine learning classification, 70
Machine Learning (ML), 20, 43–45, 50, 98
MLCA agent, 105, 125, 127–133
MLOps, 98, 99
Mobile Health (mHealth), 48
Molecular testing, 8, 21, 38
Multidisciplinary Team (MDT), 127, 132–134, 139
Multimodal AI, 57, 62, 134
Multimodal AI fusion, 57
Multi-omics integration, 66, 67, 69, 71, 72, 82, 93

N
Natural Language Processing (NLP), 43–45, 47
Non-Small Cell Lung Cancer (NSCLC), 14–16, 21, 25, 26, 28, 30, 31, 33–40, 47, 48, 50, 65, 114, 121

O
Object-oriented design, 129
Optuna, 70

P
Patient features, 98
Pembrolizumab, 39, 68, 81, 82, 86, 93, 94
Performance benchmarking, 61
PET scan, 7, 29
Pharmacogenomics, 67, 69, 71, 91, 93, 94
Prognosis, 7, 9, 14, 15, 21, 23, 26, 35, 49, 50, 67, 76, 78
Pulmonary nodule detection, 47

R
Radiation therapy, 2, 9, 26, 33, 34, 39, 50
Random forest, 44, 47, 66, 70, 72, 73, 86
Risk factors, 3, 4, 6, 7, 16, 18, 21, 30, 46, 98–102
Risk stratification, 44, 46, 51, 78, 94, 99, 127, 133, 134, 136

S
Self-Supervised Learning (SSL), 57, 58, 62
SHAP, 60, 71, 74, 87, 89, 112
Small Cell Lung Cancer (SCLC), 14–16, 21, 25, 26, 30–36, 38–40, 50
Smoking status, 85, 86, 97–99
SpO, 99, 102

Squamous cell carcinoma, 4, 8, 14, 26, 48, 107, 111, 113, 120, 136, 137, 139, 140
Stereotactic Body Radiotherapy (SBRT), 36, 37
Streamlit, 86, 87, 98, 108, 129–133
Survival analysis, 66–71, 76, 94

T
Targeted therapy, 2, 5, 8, 10, 15, 21, 25, 28, 33, 35, 37, 65, 66, 81, 91, 93
The Cancer Genome Atlas (TCGA), 66–68, 76, 77
TNM classification, 31
Tobacco smoking, 6, 16
Tumour Mutational Burden (TMB), 68, 71, 80, 81, 86, 87, 91, 92
Two-stage pipeline, 132

U
Unified CT-Based Lung Cancer Imaging Foundation (UCLIF), 56, 57, 62

V
VGG16, 130, 133, 139
Vision transformer, 45, 48, 59, 93

X
XGBoost, 44, 70–74, 86, 87, 93, 98–100

GPSR Compliance
The European Union's (EU) General Product Safety Regulation (GPSR) is a set of rules that requires consumer products to be safe and our obligations to ensure this.

If you have any concerns about our products, you can contact us on

ProductSafety@springernature.com

In case Publisher is established outside the EU, the EU authorized representative is:

Springer Nature Customer Service Center GmbH
Europaplatz 3
69115 Heidelberg, Germany

www.ingramcontent.com/pod-product-compliance
Ingram Content Group UK Ltd.
Pitfield, Milton Keynes, MK11 3LW, UK
UKHW022004280926
476074UK00003B/19
* 9 7 8 3 0 3 2 2 9 6 1 4 6 *